Old Law, New Medicine

Medical ethics and human rights

SHEILA McLEAN

An imprint of Rivers Oram Press
London and New York

First published in 1999 by Pandora, an imprint of
Rivers Oram Publishers Limited
144 Hemingford Road, London N1 1DE

Distributed in the USA by
New York University Press
Elmer Holmes Bobst Library
70 Washington Square South
New York NY10012-1091

Set in Perpetua by NJ Design Associates, Romsey, Hants
and printed in Great Britain by T.J.International (Padstow) Ltd

British Library Cataloguing in Publication Data
A catalogue record for this book is available from the British Library

ISBN 0 86358 403 9 (cloth)
ISBN 0 86358 402 0 (paperback)

To loved ones, friends, colleagues, students and Cara

Contents

Acknowledgments

The ideas in this book have taken a long time in maturation. I have been involved in teaching and researching in this area for more than twenty years, and am therefore indebted to a large number of people whose contributions have helped to shape my views. It would be invidious to single out any one academic writer who has more influenced my thinking over the years, but I would imagine those who have been most influential will become obvious to the reader. Also, in all my years of teaching I have been stimulated and challenged by many of my undergraduate and postgraduate students, and of course by my colleagues in Medical Law at Glasgow University. To them I express a debt of gratitude, although I retain sole responsibility for any criticisms which may be levelled at my approach. My parents and friends have, as always, been an enormous support, as have Sara Dunn and Katherine Bright-Holmes.

Preface

When the World Health Organisation defined health as a matter which incorporated more than just the absence of disease, it was to provoke a heated and lengthy debate. Just as the foundations of the National Health Service in the United Kingdom depended on the interaction of medical provision with other social services in the attainment of 'health', so too the WHO acknowledged that the ills which beset us may derive from a variety of social, political and economic constraints which may or may not have anything to do with our medical condition. Although the WHO definition has been subject to much criticism, it is implicit in this book that it proposed an ideological approach to health as a matter of social functioning which has much to commend it. The translation of dissatisfaction into illness, the tendency to turn to medicine for 'cure' of social or economic dysfunction, have, this book will argue, done us no favours. There are several reasons for this contention.

The first is that the Western world's use of medicine is in itself dysfunctional, in that it hands over authority to one group of professionals whose undoubted skills are nonetheless sometimes inappropriate to the resolution of the perceived problem. In this way, human problems and human values become medicalised. That is, they become compartmentalised within a specific, and it is suggested inappropriate, framework which applies its own ethics, etiquette, biases and intuitions. Thus, rather than empowering people to argue for radical social or political change, grievances are subsumed into the concept of illness. In addition, important and fundamental matters of human rights become shrouded in the mystique of the modern medical leviathan — technologised and neutralised. Moreover, one further and important consequence flows from this. No matter one's views on the law, it remains the most powerful vehicle by which fundamental change can be brought about and in it lies the power to vindicate human rights. Yet, the law's traditional deference to medicine means that, when issues are seen as medical, the individual is disenfranchised.

There are, of course, always changes in the law while a book is being prepared. It was not thought necessary to add each and every new case to this book on revision because, I hope, the argument remains sound. However, since this manuscript was originally delivered, one trend does seem worthy of comment.

In Chapter 3, I discuss the extent to which medicine has changed the face of pregnancy and reproductive liberty, by contributing to the perception that foetuses are beings with rights which may conflict with the rights of the pregnant women. In that chapter, the law is castigated for being less than proactive in protecting the freedom of women to make mature, even if regrettable, decisions about, for example, whether or not to agree to surgical intervention in the interests of their foetus. Since that chapter was written, there has been one glimmer of hope that UK law may be prepared to intervene in the interest of the woman rather than the foetus. In the case of *St George's Healthcare National Health Service Trust* v. *S* (also referred to as *Regina* v. *Collins and Others Ex parte S*),[1] a woman was given leave to sue for compensation on the basis that she had been wrongly dealt with as suffering from a mental illness and therefore deemed incompetent to reject a caesarean section. Although clearly — for the woman concerned — the award of damages could scarcely make up for the assault allegedly committed, and although this case hinged on its own particular facts and may not therefore be universalisable, nonetheless there is some reason for muted rejoicing to be found in the Court of Appeal's judgement. Indeed, this case both highlights the reluctance of the law to interfere (in the first place) and the benefits that can flow from a proactive legal approach to decisions which are described as medical, but which actually disguise agendas which have too often in the past trumped those of the individual concerned.

It would be wrong, however, to read this book as an attack on medicine or its values. Rather, the argument is based on the hypothesis that over-deference to medicine (in particular to the scientific aspect of medicine) is dangerously rights-reducing. When coupled with a legal establishment reluctant to challenge medical decision-making — indeed, apparently oblivious to the question as to whether or not doctors' decisions are inevitably about medical matters — the individual's rights to self-determination and autonomy are eroded. It is this last issue with which this book is most concerned. No matter the benevolence of the intention of doctors or courts, no matter even that their conclusions may intuitively satisfy large percentages of public opinion, if we lose a rights-based perspective on humanity we sacrifice too much. It is the job of all of us to examine carefully which are the values we most treasure, and ultimately the responsibility of the state — as often as not through the medium of the law — to resist the too easy elision of the human into the clinical. I hope that this short book makes some contribution to clarification of these responsibilities.

Introduction

In recent years, the interaction between law and medicine has become the focus of sharp, critical and analytical interest.

A society bred into challenge as opposed to acquiescence, the rapid developments in medicine and science and an apparently exponential growth in media interest in issues which can broadly be described as being about physical or mental well-being have ensured such matters a place in the spotlight. Superimposed upon this, particularly in the latter half of this century, has been the gradual gathering into the discrete ambit of one professional — the doctor — of an ever-widening range of human issues. It is to the doctor that we turn for a cure for all ills — social, political, emotional and physical.

Although much of this is probably inadvertent, it is also a feature of all professional groups that the more they widen their scope the more they avoid built-in obsolescence. The need for orthodox medicine, as well as its power, is in part predicated on how much we value its contribution. The more it offers us the miracles of creating life in a petri dish or resurrecting those who would otherwise be dead, the more the power is enhanced and the more dependent we become.

With dependence comes disenfranchisement. We may resent being infantilised, but at the same time we hand over to the clinician the right and the responsibility to decide. Without a healthy scepticism, and in the absence of an informed debate, the process of empowering this profession can only continue. Moreover, in an increasingly secular Western world, the temptation to trust — indeed the **need** to trust — some body of people who are almost magical in what they appear to be able to achieve is ever stronger. In the modern Western world, this body of people is made up of scientists/doctors.

Whether the contemporary physician likes it or not, he/she wields enormous power. Even in a world where people are more likely to challenge, and where litigation is growing apace, the group most respected remains the clinicians. We may cavil, complain and contradict but we remain in thrall ultimately to those who have the capacity to make us better, to improve us or to control our distressing symptoms. Despite the debate about the contribution orthodox medicine has actually made to human well-being, the need to believe in someone, especially someone who is in general as trustworthy as the physician, is sufficiently strong to consign doubt to the waste-basket of our minds. When we are sick, we don't want to analyse or criticise the role of the doctor — we want the doctor.

Yet, there are a large number of areas in which the doctor's role is, necessarily, ambiguous. No matter the quality of the medicine practised, and no matter the doubts of doctors themselves about the appropriateness of their involvement, human life is increasingly medicalised. In part, this is the result of the growing professionalism of medicine, in part it is our responsibility for asking too much of doctors. In part, however, it is also because the buffer which might be expected to stand between medicalisation and human rights — namely the law — has proved unwilling, unable or inefficient when asked to adjudicate on or control issues which are at best tangentially medical.

It is, of course, possible to argue that law is essentially a reactive discipline. The speed with which medicine develops, by this argument, would inevitably mean that the role of the law would simply be to adjudicate on interests already arguably breached. As a trend-setter, the law would have no role to play. However, there are three things which this book seeks to say in answer to this view of the law and legal process.

The first is that law is also a proactive medium. The fact that lawyers and legislators are not routinely trained in science or medicine should not be relevant to the way in which judgements are made. Rather, the law can set the standards which meet the challenges posed by the present and the future by thinking about the underpinning principles which are timeless and context free. It would be sufficient were appropriate tests in place against which standards are judged, and these do not require specialist clinical skills. Second, the law can be expected to be disinterested. That is, it is not appropriate for the impression to be given that one group — in this case, doctors — is apparently given special treatment. Finally, the scientific areas which have not yet been subject to rigorous legal scrutiny — such as those which are posed by the 'new' genetics — can and should be seen as issues of human rights in which the law might be expected to have both a particular interest and a specific expertise.

Simply put, the theme of this book is that matters of human rights are increasingly medicalised, rendering them vulnerable to unsuitable methods of decision-making and disempowering the populace. Currently, the law does not fulfil a proactive, rigorous and disinterested function in the way in which it deals with these matters. The aspirations of the public, encouraged by charters, by democracy and propelled by consumerism, are destined to be frustrated. Increasingly, what we want is what we are told is available. The language of power is a mere obfuscation of what is really happening. Our right to participate actively in our lives and our futures is minimised by the deference to the social and professional role of others. The one vehicle — the law — to which we are forced to turn for vindication of our rights, our hopes and our expectations, is sufficiently subjugated to those whom we wish to challenge, that frustration of ambitions is the likely outcome.

What this book does not do is to criticise doctors, lawyers or any other group. Its aim is to expose the often inadvertent collusion between two of the major powers in contemporary society. It is intended to ask rather than answer questions. If it is profoundly disagreed with it will have succeeded as much as if every reader agreed with every word.

1 Setting the Scene

In the novel *Jurassic Park* the scientist, Ian Malcolm, has this to say:

> Ever since Newton and Descartes, science has explicitly offered us the vision of total control. Science has claimed the power to eventually control everything, through its understanding of natural laws. But in the twentieth century, that claim has been shattered beyond repair ... And so the grand vision of science, hundreds of years old — the dream of total control — has died, in our century. And with it much of the justification, the rationale for science to do what it does. And for us to listen to it.[1]

Even given this assertion, we still **do** listen to science — even revere it. In particular, we listen to doctors. The translation of medicine from an art into a science, with its plethora of techniques and technologies, dominates the human condition in the twentieth century. Increasingly individuals and communities turn to the physician to provide reassurance and affirmation — reassurance of a future and affirmation of health or ill-health. We cling to an intuitive understanding of when we are or are not functioning adequately, and when we feel that functioning is impaired, it is as often as not to the doctor that we turn for assistance.

The extent to which medicine has been successful in shaping our world can be seen by the number of people who turn to it for assistance. In 1987, for example, the UK Government Report 'Promoting Better Health'[2] showed just how substantial the role played by medicine and related professions was in the daily life of the community.

> On an average working day, about $3/4$ million people see their family doctor and about the same number get medicines on prescription from their local pharmacist. About 300,000 go to the dentist. At least 100,000 are visited by nurses or other health professionals working in the community. Around 70,000 attend community health clinics and 40,000 have their sight tested. Over £5,000 million a year is spent on primary care.[3]

And this estimate takes no account of the number of people currently in hospital.

Health and its provision are political issues in all countries. In the United States President Clinton's proposed health-care reform, designed to expand access, was possibly one of the most fiercely debated issues of his Presidency. Scarcely surprising when about 14 per cent of the US gross domestic product is spent on health care.[4] Yet, as Schwartz points out 'the increased amount of our resources devoted to health care ... and the consistently high levels of those people not covered by even that very high expenditure — 15 per cent across the United States, and up to 25 per cent in some states — have made the system unacceptable. To put it simply, the cost of health care and the widespread lack of access to it have become a national scandal.'[5]

This is not the place to delve into the quagmire that is the debate about resource allocation, but the intense argument about the availability of resources both at national and individual levels is one which serves as part of the backdrop to the theme of this book.

The reason for the debate, to be sure, is the apparently inevitable differential between supply and demand in the provision of health care services. The premise is that everything which doctors believe to be within their purview is truly a matter of health care, and must therefore ideally be met from the health-care budget.

Despite the 'miracles' of modern medicine, of course, much of what we seek from clinicians is truly beyond their capacities. Indeed, some would argue that medicine has had a remarkably limited impact on the health status of the individual, and others, for example Illich, would go even further, claiming that 'The medical establishment has become a major threat to health'.[6] Even if we don't agree with Illich it is clear that the transformation of medicine into a science has had profound effects at a number of levels. Not least, it has forced the doctor into a particular role within particular Western societies. The contemporary conviction that science, and therefore medicine, are value-free and sophisticated disciplines may have paradoxical effects. As Illich points out, 'The radical monopoly over health care that the contemporary physician claims now forces him to reassume priestly and royal functions that his ancestors gave up when they became specialised as technical healers.'[7] In addition, the claims made for medicine also mean that the decision-making power vested in those who profess it has widened considerably — some would say inappropriately — and is often not subject to external control.

Neither the fact that a discipline is scientific nor the professionalism and technical expertise of those with the relevant knowledge justifies a lack of scrutiny from non-scientific perspectives. Like all human endeavours, technology and its application are value-laden enterprises: they must be tested against values such as compassion which emerge from culture, or principles like justice which as societies we claim to endorse. Much of this book will be concerned with precisely this kind of testing. But first it is necessary to clarify the nature of the agents at the centre of the discussion — namely medicine and those who practice it.

We all accept that medical practitioners are in the business of health, but we lack an adequate description of what health is. A satisfactory definition of health has even eluded the World Health Organisation.[8] There is, therefore, immense scope for any apparent malfunction in the life of an individual to be categorised as ill-health, and for the doctor to be seen as the person with both capacity and authority to resolve it. As Kennedy notes 'the scope of the alleged unique competence of the doctor has become as wide, as imprecise and as flexible as the meanings given to the notions of health and ill health'.[9]

In this scenario, all ills, social, personal, societal and global, can somehow be refashioned, neutralised, even eradicated, by the miracles generated by the modern religion that is medical science. The power to dispense its goods is vested in its priests — namely physicians. This leads to the inclusion of much of the human condition within the medical model. For example, as Anleu points out, 'Medical intervention in the area of conception suggests that infertility is a disease or an illness' justifying its control by doctors.[10] Yet, 'Infertility has not always been a medical category. The activities of the medical profession, particularly the segments of obstetrics and gynaecology, have been instrumental in its designation as a medical condition requiring medical treatment and intervention. Medicine is oriented to locating and identifying illness by creating social meanings of illness where such interpretations previously were absent.'[11]

However, much of what people demand — and get — from medicine is non-medical, and a culture which turns to the doctor as a latter-day Messiah, will be one which places exceptional demands on health-care budgets. But it will also be more than this. Failure to address the question as to whether or not the doctor is the appropriate decision-maker, or has the requisite skills to resolve a perceived problem, perpetuates both resource problems and the identification of all decisions made by doctors as being medical ones.

Illich's views may be too extreme for many, but there is a certain resonance in his claim that:

> Iatrogenic medicine reinforces a morbid society in which social control of the population by the medical system turns into a principal economic activity. It serves to legitimise social arrangements into which many people do not fit. It labels the disabled as unfit and breeds a new category of patients. People who are angered, sickened, and impaired by their industrial labour and leisure can escape only into a life under medical supervision and are thereby seduced or disqualified from political struggle for a healthier world.[12]

Much of what we expect, aspire to, need or choose is seen as dependent on our state of health, however defined. The guardians of that health have enormous power and their status as scientists reinforces their position as the new meritocracy. Authority is often uncritically invested in the physician at the expense of personal responsibility and power. The physicians' role therefore expands, as new phenomena are absorbed into their domain of competence. Thus, the question of what is properly a medical matter is obfuscated by the patina of certainty presented by orthodox medicine. So, as will be seen later, decisions about quality of life are substantially handed over by the law to the physician. Yet the decisions rest on a complex mix of values, intuitions and opinion, as well as on scientific criteria, not typically associated with medical practitioners, whose views are revered substantially, because they are seen to be scientific and therefore 'right'. Realistically, of course, the practice of medicine is an amalgam of science and art, yet, as Katz points out, 'What is disturbing ... is that physicians are so reluctant to acknowledge to themselves and their patients which of their opinions are based on science and which on intuition'.[13]

Moreover, the task of medicine — identifying and caring for the sick — can present a jaundiced view of the community as a whole. Mechanic says, 'to the extent that medical care identifies more illness, sustains life among chronically ill persons, and allows the survival of persons with congenital and other defects, it contributes to higher levels of recognized morbidity and disability in the population'.[14]

The increasing classification of illness and disability among the population does have generalised political impact, but it also affects the individual directly. The emphasis on dysfunction (physical or mental) as a predictor of the capacity to engage in the community serves to enhance the vulnerability of the individual. Medicine, as responsible for 'health', becomes both increasingly respected and astonishingly powerful. As Illich says, 'Society has transferred to physicians the exclusive right to determine what constitutes sickness, who is or might become sick, and what shall be done to such people'.[15] In a world where the perception of health is so central to social, political and personal intercourse, this is an awe-inspiring power indeed.

Wittingly or unwittingly the physician holds the key to the well-being of every individual citizen, at least in the Western world. Given the power to define their own terms, doctors then also stand as moral gatekeepers to the services which only they apparently can provide.

It must also be recognised that the power of the professional who apparently has a monopoly on the answers devalues other options and groups. It is important to note the extent to which the professionalisation of medicine has acted to produce monopoly and to neutralise the possibility of alternative coping strategies. Turner argues that the former 'can be seen as an occupational strategy to maintain certain monopolistic privileges and rewards'.[16] Commending the efficiency of the medical profession for having 'been relatively successful in maintaining its position within the class structure and the professional hierarchy over the last 100 years by regulating and controlling access to health care delivery'.[17] he notes that 'One important function ... of medical dominance is to preserve and extend the medical access to its clientele by limiting and subordinating adjacent occupations.'[18]

Coping mechanisms which go beyond and challenge the adoption of the sick role and the (too often almost automatic) pharmacological fix are subverted by the expectations fostered by clinicians. Illich would claim that this is an inevitable disabling feature of advanced industrial society which, he claims is 'sick-making because it disables people from coping with their environment and, when they break down, it substitutes a "clinical" prosthesis for the broken relationships. People would rebel against such an environment if medicine did not explain their biological disorientation as a defect in their health, rather than as a defect in the way of life which is imposed on them or which they impose on themselves.'[19]

Evidence of the use of medical diagnosis as a bandage for the spiritually, socially and politically wounded abounds. Medicine knows what it can do but it may not know why it does it or whether doing it is right.

We would do well to reflect on Pellegrino's exposition of the extent to which culture is inextricably linked to the ethos of medicine. As he says:

The dominant characteristics of Western science, ethics, and politics are mutually supportive. Western science is

empirical and experimental, pursuing objectivity and quan-
tification of experience. Ultimately it attempts to control
nature to the greatest extent possible. Western ethics is
analytical, rationalistic, dialectical, and often secular in spirit.
Western politics is liberal, democratic, and individualistic
and governed by law. Western science, ethics, and politics
provide an environment that gives rise to and sustains the
use of complex medical technologies. As a result, it is difficult to divorce medical knowledge and the benefits it offers
from the Western cultural and ethical milieu that support
and sustain them.[20]

Yet the impact of the Western tradition of medicine is not a
matter of indifference to other cultures. Global enterprises such
as the trade in pharmaceuticals and the Human Genome Project
also invade other cultures whose traditions are equally valued but
may ultimately be threatened. The pharmaceutical fix disvalues
traditional healing. The reduction of people to a collection of their
genes flies in the face of traditional religious and ethical perspectives of the soul. Value systems vary, with no one arguably having
an overwhelming claim to the right, yet 'as the power and influence of medical science and technology grow, these conflicting
systems of belief will be drawn into more acute confrontation and
conflict with each other'.[21]

Medicine, therefore, cohabits comfortably with the political and
ethical dialectic of society. Its values mirror those of a technological age and its rationales are seldom subject to question. To
this extent, it can pose enormous challenges to the place of the
individual in a community. Medicine first defines its own competence, then finds clinical answers to the questions it itself has posed.
Finally, it decides who shall benefit from its capacities or be
subject to its experiments.

The vision of medicine as a science reinforces our subjugation to it. Science is thought to be rational, value-free and accurate. A scientific solution removes the need for personal responsibility while at the same time obfuscating the real issues facing humanity. Science it is that has pursued policies of eugenics (in tandem with political will), assisted reproduction, the search for a genetic explanation of social characteristics and the quest for control of life and death. Moreover, medical science's rapidly expanding technologies bring their own inherent and complex ethical and social questions and what medicine discovers can lead to personal confusion about what it is to be an individual in a given community.

The question may be posed, however, whether this is anything about which we, as ordinary citizens, should be concerned. Perhaps we have chosen the future ourselves and are prepared to wrestle with the dilemmas that choice poses in the interests of the advances and benefits which are undoubtedly on offer. But how realistic is this view? Quite apart from the logical impossibility of ordinary people truly being this informed, there are underlying — and vital — choices made totally outside the control of the individual citizen. As Kass has said:

> Introduction of new technologies often appears to be the result of no decision whatsoever, or of the culminations of decisions too small or unconscious to be recognised as such. Fate seems to hold the reins: What can be done is done. But technological advance is not automatic. Someone is deciding on the basis of some notions of desirability, no matter how self-serving or altruistic.[22]

Somewhere decisions are made that certain goals are worth pursuing — for example in developing the techniques of in vitro fertilisation — but it is certain that they are not made by us, nor is the motive for their development clear. However, once commenced, the right to control them is vested in those who manipulate the science, and — every bit as important — they come to form part of the medical empire. Nonetheless, we might feel that there is nothing inherently wrong in progress being determined by those who, after all, have the technical knowledge which we lack. In any event, surely in a democracy, we have the capacity to control what happens next?

But it is not really that simple. It is a mistake to believe that either the possession or the use of technical knowledge is value neutral. As Pellegrino and Thomasma warn, 'Without the reasonable restraints imposed by philosophical critique, medicine and its practitioners may unintentionally convert science and medical method into a muddled philosophy of human life'.[23] And given that we all accept that advance brings with it new moral dilemmas, there is no evidence, empirical or otherwise, which would lead to the conclusion that those driving the science are any better than anyone else at identifying, analysing and resolving these important issues.

The belief that democratic systems inevitably devolve actual power to individuals is one which is at least arguable where powerful monopolies both shape and control the debate. The likely fact that the majority of a given community has great faith in modern medicine and believes that it is best left to the doctors should not preclude a rational critique. No matter how small or sporadic are the voices raised in challenge against the juggernaut of medicalisation, and no matter if the majority is satisfied, there must always be a place for an exposition of the presumptions which underlie the power which mere majority may seem to provide.[24]

Healthy cynicism about the extent to which power should uncritically be devolved to any one group or discipline forms the central platform of this book. The underlying matters of concern are issues of human rights. No discipline and no individual has, or should have, the power to strip others of their liberty to reach out for their aspirations or to stake their legitimate claims. The danger is that human rights take second place to the paternalism or monopolisation of one group substantially because they can claim scientific reasoning as their bedrock. The location of power, then, is critical as is the need to address the human rights issues which underlie the distribution of that power. In liberal democracies, the notion that power can or should be exercised unfettered by constraints and accountability is anathema. It follows, therefore, that mechanisms must be in place which have both the authority and the will to undertake rational scrutiny both of the enterprise and of those who carry it out. These mechanisms must address the underlying distinctiveness of the ventures they assess as well as bearing in mind the principles which lie at the heart of the need for control in the first place.

The boundaries of any discipline's method will play a significant part in the process of scrutiny and the consequences of its use. As Franklin puts it: 'Science is an endeavour that separates knowledge from experience. That is both the glory of science and its greatest drawback because in many ways science finds it impossible to bring experience back into the newly acquired knowledge. As a consequence, we now have to struggle with the application of non-contextual scientific knowledge to the very context-bound problem of human rights.'[25]

And this exposes the nub of the problem. The attempt to translate content into context is one which must be made externally to the discipline itself, and with prominence given to the rights of those whose lives are affected by the decision reached. The assumption of scientific superiority is not in se erroneous, but the consequence which too often flows from it is. That the average citizen, the legislator or the judge generally lacks the knowledge of the doctor is no justification for evading the issue of rights. As Katz says, 'The history of the physician–patient relationship from ancient times to the present bears testimony to physicians' caring dedication to their patients' physical welfare. The same history, by its account of the silence that has pervaded this relationship, also bears testimony to physicians' inattention to their patients' right and need to make their own decisions.'[26]

Failure to conceptualise what is going on in terms of human rights leads to individual disempowerment. Medicine can certainly try to deal with the diseases which most concern us, but it can also absorb social and personal problems into its own unique sphere of influence. As Kennedy has pointed out, 'failure to examine the question [as to what is a medical decision] has resulted in decisions being taken by doctors which may not properly be within the unique or special competence of a doctor qua doctor to make'.[27]

Medicalisation, then, has the potential to threaten or infringe human rights. The time has never been more ripe for a clear investigation of this issue. The control exercised over our lives and lifestyles by the incorporation of scientific values into the centre of our judgements, individual and collective, has never been more intense. The increasing technical gap between the individual and the scientist/doctor serves further to distance those about whom decisions are made from those who actually make them. The exercise of power becomes at once more subtle and less accountable. This suggests no deliberate conspiratorial phenomenon but rather points to the fact that subtle shifts in social perception and relationships can lead to situations in which the traditional guardians of accountability, for example the law, are muted or neutered.' Franklin puts this problem starkly, saying 'One of the important aspects of modern technological practice is that it allows the control of people in ways that make the control invisible. No longer does Big Brother blare out of loud speakers. Big Brother barely beeps today. The invisibility of control ought to concern us very profoundly.'[28]

The next question, therefore, must be — how do we wrest control into our own hands? Traditionally, Western societies have looked to the law to achieve this function. McVeigh and Wheeler see law as still having 'a powerful ordering role in almost all regulation ...',[29] even if they also feel that, 'As a dominant language of social organisation, law has been of declining importance since the eighteenth century'.[30] Despite the debate about the relationship between law and morality, it is contended here that at least some law either shapes, determines or reflects commonly agreed and acceptable principles. It might well be expected, therefore, that in areas so important to the good functioning of the individual and the state as the control of health, even of life and death, the law could be relied on for the kind of disinterested decision-making which would serve to balance interests appropriately, and vindicate rights unequivocally.

But this is not in fact the case: both our society and our law seem happy enough to pass the burden of decision-making on many moral (or at least non-clinical) matters to the clinician (whether or not the clinician actually wants to accept this load). Decisions about who should live and who should die are perhaps the starkest examples of choices which are value-laden and complex. Medical progress certainly contributes to the creation of these questions in the first place, but it can scarcely claim a monopoly of the answers since they touch the very core of our ethical and moral codes.

An apparently unarguable assertion this may be, but it is one, in fact, which is more honoured in the breach than in its observance. The rhetoric that accepts that decisions are bigger than merely clinical ones already stands discomfited by the control over sensitive ethical problems which has in reality been seized by medicine. For example, pre-implantation and pre-natal screening and diagnosis openly seek to prevent the birth of 'defective' children. Selective non-treatment of disabled infants ensures that the 'survival of the fittest' is given a (not very) gentle clinical nudge. Decisions to withhold or withdraw therapy when these result in death are much bigger questions than the merely clinical, yet they are often handed over on the flimsiest of justifications to the medical profession. The (UK) *Report of the Select Committee on Medical Ethics*,[31] which addressed the questions raised at the end of life, shows just how readily such decisions are accommodated. The report acknowledges that, 'Some people may consider that our conclusions overall give too much weight to the role of accepted medical practice, and that we advocate leaving too much responsibility in the hands of doctors and other members of the health-care team. They may argue that doctors and their colleagues are no better qualified than any other group of people to take ethical decisions about life and death which ultimately have a bearing not only on individual patients but on society as a whole.'[32] They may indeed!

But, the same report concludes, 'no other group of people is better qualified to do so. Doctors and their colleagues are versed in what is medically possible, and are therefore best placed to evaluate the likely outcomes of different courses of action in the very different circumstances of each individual case. By virtue of their vocation, training and professional integrity they may be expected to act with rectitude and compassion.'[33] But this does not justify them in monopolising the 'right' decisions in any issue beyond those within their professional remit. In other words, they are uniquely qualified to reach a medical prognosis, but the outcome of that prognosis is a matter which has moral, ethical, social and political consequences which doctors' training and technical knowledge in no way equip them to address, far less to answer.

There is also a legal consequence of this abandonment of morality to medicine. Decisions which are deemed to be medical will be assessed for their legal standing by using the tests traditionally applied to matters of professional practice. In virtually all Western jurisdictions, albeit with some variation in emphasis, this means that the physician's behaviour will be tested not against an abstract set of ethical principles, nor even against its effect on human rights, but rather against what other doctors believe to be correct or appropriate.[34] In other words, matters of fundamental ethical values are at the mercy of professional practice and etiquette.

A second major consequence of medicalisation is the reduction of humanity to 'collections of organ systems and deposits of disease entities'.[35] If we are to recognise and value the unique potential of every human being we must surely eschew this mechanistic, biological explanation. Intellectual creativity, compassion, community and humanity itself are threatened by the reductionism sometimes all too obvious in medicine and science. Scientific method undoubtedly makes a valuable contribution to an explanation of part of what it is to be human but it is by no means sufficient per se to uncover more than a small part of life's mysteries. As was hinted earlier, not just the deification of the scientist, but also the mystique of scientific thinking (rational, clear and value-free) have profoundly affected contemporary Western societies and — if given inappropriate prominence — can serve to stunt the individual's sense of self and to limit the potential for moral growth.

In the face of advances in genetics, in the light of the incorporation of more and more human conditions into the sphere of medicine, we are right to stop and consider whether our relatively uncritical acceptance of the role of medicine has not gone too far. The reduction of the human being to a set of predetermined characteristics finally removes all hope of change, of expansion, of value. Just as gender and race became for many an acceptable basis for mindless characterisation and failure to value individuals, so too what science is now seeking to find out about our genetic make-up may provide the basis for clinical discrimination.

At the heart of this book lies the belief that freedom and dignity can indeed be protected against the unwitting presumptions of the modern gurus, and that the best protection is afforded by law and legal process. Whatever role law has in relation to broadly based ethics and morality, it lays claim to internal ethics which are substantially uncontroversial and which provide what is — to date at least — the best model available. Concepts of justice, formal and distributive, due process and a tradition of respect for rights are inherent in legal systems and can provide a framework within which complex moral matters can be debated and perhaps even resolved. However, a significant and crucial caveat must be entered here. The argument is not that the law actually does this — rather that it could. Each of the topics considered will highlight the extent to which, in my view, the law has reneged on its promise when evaluating matters which are claimed as falling within the province of medicine. This is no starry-eyed attempt to justify the simple transfer of power from one group of professionals to another. The argument concedes the shortcomings of all involved, but at the same time contends that we have a suitable mechanism in existence with its own potential to render the hidden accountable and the wrong right.

This is not an anti-doctor book. It is not another sad attempt to devalue one discipline or set of individuals who are fair game because of their social and public status. It is rather an attempt to accommodate all of the good that doctors and medicine do within a critical framework which — with no disrespect — seeks to disentangle what doctors should do from what they actually do. The inevitable consequence of professionalism may be the gathering in of the widest possible competences, some of which may be inappropriate, although this is not to say that this is a desire, conscious or otherwise, of individual clinicians. And the common consequence of faith in professionals may be the apparently willing transfer of power, appropriate or otherwise, into their hands. Be that as it may, the incorporation of ethical problems within the discrete framework of medicine has many consequences, foreseen and unforeseen which must be addressed. The Human Genome Project and the consequent ability to shape reproductive and other choices, force analysis of the ways, if any, that medicine might be harnessed to maximise its potential for good and minimise its real capacity for harm.

For now, the doctor stands as both the judge of 'normality' and the gatekeeper of resources. The technological impulse or imperative has come to dominate and control both those who are indisputably ill and those whose dysfunction is social or political. It has the capacity to create new sick roles, to pit one individual against another, to refuse to lie down in the face of the inevitable and to distort the very humanity which it overtly seeks to assist. As Kass has said, 'Thoughtful men have long known that the campaign for the technological conquest of nature, conducted under the banner of modern science, would someday train its guns against the commanding officer, man himself'. [36] It is time for man (and woman) to stand up to this threat, and for this to be effective, a firm and unshakeable commitment to shared values is needed. As has been said, 'it may well be that our biggest problem lies in identifying a morality (which reaches well beyond just health care) which can form the basis of our national and global aspirations. Once achieved, however, we may find that the law becomes a more valuable weapon in a struggle with whose aims few can be in dispute.' [37]

It is not irrelevant to draw attention to these problems. It is not trivial to point to the human impact of the seizure of control of our destiny, no matter how respected and respectable those seizing it may be. It is not disrespectful to resist inappropriate classification. It is not without sense to find some sympathy with the following characterisation:

'Trust us', resonate doctors at the frequency of libertarianism. 'We are professionals, driven by our fiduciary duties to help you.' 'Grant us respect,' chant hospitals, 'for we are charities with all that implies.' 'Leave politics out of health care,' the full chorus repeats in a basso ostinato, 'for we are nonpolitical.'[38]

It is wise and productive to assert our humanity as having precedence over our clinical status. It is prudent to challenge the translation of hidden or overt professional bias into our personal and social reality. It is imperative to resist unthinking and far-reaching categorisation. To achieve these things, 'Reconciliation of advances in medicine and science with values expressed through human rights is necessary to preserve the bioethical balance; to ensure that the risks to patients, providers and the subjects of biotechnology are minimised'.[39]

Each of the chapters in this book has a number of issues in common. Most importantly, they show the ways in which the power of medicalisation can serve to disenfranchise, to minimise people's individual opportunity to come to terms with problems which are often at best tangentially clinical. Moreover, in some of the chapters, there is an underlying theme which concerns the extent to which gender may play a part in the medical response to perceived problems, or may serve as a basis for the generation of new and complex dilemmas. Fundamental to the entire argument is the claim that current legal responses (primarily, although not exclusively, judicial) are inadequate to attain the goal of the protection of human rights. The attitude of the judiciary has often obscured the real issues at stake by adopting a combination of deference to the professional and the rhetoric of individual liberties. Or, as one commentator put it,

> Judges were hesitant to intrude on medical matters, and not only for reasons of unfamiliarity with the ways in which physicians worked. Their impulse to foster individual self-determination collided with an equally strong desire to maintain the authority of the profession, both for the sake of professionals and for the 'best interests' of patients. The law had always respected the arcane expertise of physicians and rarely held them liable if they practised 'good medicine'. [40]

This is no less true today. It is not necessary to believe in conspiracy theory to make this conclusion clear. This book does not imply malice on the part of medicine or the law, not does it go so far as to suggest that there is a systematic attempt to strip individuals of power. What it does do, however, is to challenge the presumption that medicine is a morally neutral enterprise (one which is probably not shared by doctors themselves) and to assert that, at worst, individual and collective values are threatened by the continuing absorption into medicine of matters which are truly substantially if not wholly matters of human rights. In this way, people's desire to live free and self-determining lives can be threatened by being taken over and judged within an inappropriate set of ethical or professional principles.

Medicalisation of these issues can be a powerful force for coercion, and can discourage challenge by appealing to the 'scientific' or esoteric knowledge held by those who are given responsibility for decision-making about our lives. The conclusion is that the handing over of so much power to medicine is a direct threat to human freedoms and severely limits the capacity of individuals to make sense and take charge of themselves and their environment. I cannot pretend to come up with an answer by drafting a watertight alternative agenda for the law. Rather I will both recognise that, 'The role of the law ... is a complex one, in particular where health is not seen as one homogeneous, medically determined concept'[41] and argue that a radical reassessment of the role of medicine is a prerequisite for the formulation of an appropriate legal response to the challenge to human rights which we now face.

2 The Reproduction Revolution
Liberation or Liability?

The title of this chapter was carefully chosen. For too long, women were denied access to the full richness of life because of their biological capacities — defined and constrained by their reproductive functions. However, the nineteenth century saw the growth of the women's movement, whose primary platform was the struggle to control reproduction — to space the bearing of children, to reduce women's social and economic dependence on men and to save women's lives by sparing them repeated and sometimes dangerous pregnancies.[1] In some ways, the picture has now turned full circle, with much of contemporary interest being focused on assisting women to have children. The question considered here is whether or not this changed pattern has truly contributed to the liberation of women.

In particular over the last 20 years or so emphasis on fertility — or perhaps more appropriately, infertility — has re-emerged as a personal, social and political phenomenon. This revitalised interest is in large part due to the developments in science and medicine which have undoubtedly changed the landscape of infertility and offered options to those who would otherwise not have the opportunity of bearing children. In addition, the decriminalisation of abortion in certain circumstances has contributed to fanning the flames of a debate about reproductive rights and control which expands every day with developments in pre-natal diagnostic capacities and the possibility of genetic therapy. From being seen (as the Supreme Court in the United States said several decades ago)[2] as a private matter, reproductive behaviour is at the centre of a significant, and worthwhile, public debate.

It has been said that 'It is widely believed that some 10 per cent of married couples who wish to have children are unable to do so by reason of infertility ... '[3] In reality, the number of those who are for all practical purposes infertile is much greater than this, since this figure excludes those who are unable to have children as a result of the fact that they are not in a sexual relationship or because of their sexuality. Since current approaches in a number of jurisdictions tend to discourage the provision of assisted reproductive techniques to these groups,[4] their status as functionally infertile, unable to bear children or create a family, is virtually guaranteed.

Yet, the importance of procreation is unarguable for very many people. One of the pioneers of assisted reproduction, Robert Edwards, has said that 'The desire to have children must be among the most basic of human instincts and denying it can lead to considerable psychological and social difficulties'.[5] Seeking ways to circumvent infertility has become big business in medicine, since it appears that Edwards' assertion has been readily accepted, based presumably not only on the individual experiences of those who seek to develop the techniques but also on the fact that people present themselves as infertile and look for assistance.

One avenue is, of course, to explore the reasons for infertility, and it is thought that these are about equally male and female in their roots. Infertility, therefore, is not merely something which affects women. However, arguably, much more effort has been put into finding the 'answer' rather than asking the questions. The 'quick fix' of developing sophisticated techniques and technologies is more glamorous than arguing for changes in society, in the environment and in sexual practices, all of which may affect fertility.[6]

It also places control of the solution firmly in the hands of medicine, with all that this entails. And, perhaps inevitably, this has meant a concentration on the female role in reproduction. The vast majority of the new technologies are focused on the woman and her body, even if she is not the individual who is infertile.

This approach has a long history. Society is often criticised for describing women largely in terms of their reproductive capacities, and its structures are such that Woollett has suggested that 'The dilemma for childless and infertile women in this society is that the opportunities provided by motherhood and the needs it fulfils cannot readily be met elsewhere; not having a child may restrict a woman's opportunities to engage in close, intimate and long term relationships.'[7] Equally the condition of being a woman becomes pathological. For example, Ussher points out that 'The discourse of reproductive liability and vulnerability is not confined to the menstrual cycle. Pregnancy, childbirth and the postnatal period have been pathologised in the same (convenient) way, positioning women's experiences as an illness in need of intervention, and interpreting any distress or unhappiness as individual pathology.'[8] And Plato, for example, said 'The womb is an animal which longs to generate children. When it remains barren too long after puberty, it is distressed and sorely disturbed, and straying about in the body and cutting off the passages of the breath, it impedes respiration and brings the sufferer into the extremist anguish and provokes all manner of diseases besides.'[9]

However inadequate Plato's medical and social knowledge, the assumptions underlying his comments demonstrate that, from the earliest times, the hypothesis has been that childbearing or childlessness is a concern of and for women rather than men. The purpose of this chapter is to look at infertility as a social construct which is intimately bound up in our perceptions of women and what it is to be female, or a 'real woman'.

Of course, not everyone agrees with all or part of this underlying premise, and many are hostile to the radical feminist
perspective which claims that advances in reproductive technologies are yet another example of the battle for control which
exists between men and women. [10] Engelhardt, for example, in
his influential book *The Foundations of Bioethics* said 'in vitro fertilisation and techniques that will allow us to study and control human
reproduction are morally neutral instruments for the realisation
of profoundly important human goals, which are bound up with
the realisation of the good of others: children for infertile parents
and greater health for the children that will be born'. [11]

Others would dismiss the need for adopting a consequentialist approach — that is, they would discount in whole or in part
the need to scrutinise carefully the rationale behind the developments, their personal and social implications and outcomes and
would argue against a need for directive intervention in their
control. On this view, what is significant is the role of the doctor
as moral gatekeeper. The question is not so much what in totality are the implications and concerns that surround modern
reproduction but rather who should decide on what should be
done, to whom and under what circumstances. As has been said,
somewhat colourfully: 'It is not enough to show that disaster
awaits if the process is not controlled. A man walking East in Omaha
will drown in the Atlantic — if he does not stop. The argument
must also rest on the evidence about the likelihood that judgment
and control will be exercised responsibly .... Collectively we
have significant capacity to exercise judgment and control .... Our
record has been rather good in regard to medical treatment and
research.' [12]

If this were in fact the case, then arguably a number of the
concerns which I will go on to voice would take on a lesser significance. However, even a brief review of our recent history shows

that we cannot afford to make such rather self-satisfied assumptions. From Beecher's exposé in the 1960s of the unlicensed, unconsented to and occasionally untenable experimentation which was being conducted in the United States,[13] to the manipulation of reproductive liberties in the United States in the early part of this century[14] and to the pogroms of the Second World War, it cannot be said that trusting those who control technologies is either the safest or the most appropriate response. As Murray has said, 'History is rich with examples of scientific perspectives used inappropriately for political purposes'.[15] One such purpose may well be the generation of social constructs which delineate and distribute functions and values which serve to reinforce the supremacy or superiority of one group over another.

And this is particularly so when reproduction (particularly focused on women) is what is being controlled or manipulated. Before Nazi Germany engaged so wholeheartedly in compulsory sterilisation programmes, control of fertility was a major political issue in other countries, perhaps most notably the United States.[16] Immigration laws were changed in the face of 'evidence' that people from Mediterranean countries were biologically inferior. The first President Roosevelt famously threatened the genesis of a Black America given higher birth rates in that community. Elementary genetic information — perhaps one should say guesswork — led to the belief that certain characteristics, such as criminality, were inherited. The outcome of this was the putting in place of laws which authorised the compulsory sterilisation of certain groups and hundreds of thousands of people (mostly women) were accordingly sterilised against their will or without their knowledge and consent.[17] As an aside, it is worth noting that such eugenic programmes were supported by a wide range of political affiliations, and even by Marie Stopes who is usually remembered as a pioneer of the women's movement!

Even against the backdrop of a written Constitution guaranteeing rights and freedoms, the Supreme Court of the United States, whose responsibility it is to interpret the Constitution, declared such laws to be constitutional, most famously in the case of *Buck v. Bell*[18] concluding that 'three generations of imbeciles are enough.'[19] In this case Carrie Buck challenged the constitutionality of a law which allowed the Superintendent of the institution in which she lived to authorise her sterilisation against her will. The evidence used to support the sterilisation concerned allegations that Carrie Buck and her mother were both 'feebleminded' and that she had a child with similar intellectual limitations. This evidence was, of course, designed to show the hereditary nature of the condition and to vindicate the non-consensual operation. Interestingly, it later emerged that the child had not been tested and was not in fact mentally disabled. The production of this evidence was, however, a little late for Carrie Buck.

Reproduction, therefore, is not simply a merely private matter, and this is particularly so when third parties — in the case of assisted reproduction, doctors — are involved in it. As is the case in all spheres of life, those who control the technology have considerable power. As Sherwin says,

> Because effective forms of reproductive technology increase the possibilities for human intervention in reproduction, they create opportunities for greater power in the hands of whoever controls that technology. Throughout history, those who have been in positions of power and authority have sought to exercise their power over the sexual and reproductive lives of the less powerful: for example, amongst the powers that Plato reserved for the philosopher-kings of the republic was the authority to arrange the reproductive pairings for all classes.[20]

Thus she continues: 'Although the new reproductive technologies can provide individuals with greater power to determine their own procreative choices, actual control may belong to others.'[21]

And this is a highly significant point. Simplistically, it might seem unarguable that the new technologies **do** offer increased choice. But, even leaving aside the fact that the technologies are by no means freely available and that 'choice' may, therefore, be restricted to those who can afford it, a real choice demands an element of control. Control, albeit not necessarily in the sense of the technical, is predicated on the availability of information and the power to contribute to the ways in which services are offered and organised. But the technologies which appear to facilitate choice are, or have been, largely in the control of men, even if they primarily affect, or are carried out on, women. This, therefore, is an area ripe for discourse which is broadly speaking feminist. As Hammer and Allen put it: 'Reproduction engineering ... is almost entirely in the hands of men, as are the governmental and voluntary agencies that fund this research and the decision-makers in the companies that will commercially exploit these scientific findings, reaping large profits.'[22]

It must be said at this stage that neither the purpose nor the intention of this chapter is to minimise or make judgements upon any individual or group of individuals and their reproductive decisions — whether they are to have or not to have children. Rather, it is designed to describe an alternative view of what we think we are doing when we make decisions about reproduction, and hopefully to do so constructively. The perspective which I will address begins, in view of what has gone before, by describing reproductive decision-making from what might broadly be described as a feminist position. However, it must be remembered that feminist arguments do not simply take one homogeneous or even extreme position. For my purposes, arguments will be described as feminist when they take the woman to be the central character in the debate. Thus, they may be made by men or women. I take this position because it is often under-represented, and yet as an aspect of the history of society as a whole, and women's place in it in particular, it cannot be dismissed as irrelevant or peripheral. The central character in assisted reproduction is the woman. In other words it is legitimate social comment. Moreover, it serves to address starkly the premise of this entire book — namely that medicalisation of human matters can, and often does, provide a platform for reducing liberty, wittingly or unwittingly.

The combination of assumptions about individuals or groups with the power of medicine is seldom more acutely evident than in matters of reproduction. Since continuing the species is vital, and is still seen as 'women's work', a great deal can be learned from the way in which medicine controls women's reproductive desires and capacities. Feminist theory is both a comment on, and a reflection of, the kind of society in which we live. That is to say those who see women as potentially or actually manipulated by reproductive technology are aware of, and sympathetic to, the desire to have children — indeed, many of the major figures in that group will be parents themselves. What they are **concerned** about is the extent to which infertile women are potentially being pressurised by a system which reflects values which they would see as male-dominated, or are being offered apparent choices which may seem to be liberating but which are in fact designed to reinforce a stereotype of women which has profound consequences for the other contributions which they have to make to the community. As one commentator (male) has said in a different context: 'Feminist critics of the new reproductive technologies have shown how difficult it is to divorce these technologies from their ideological contexts'.[23]

What is **not** true is that these writers and commentators do not care about infertility and those who are affected by it — rather their approach to the issues is different. As Gena Corea, a leading feminist writer, says:

> The suffering infertility causes women is enormous and deserves to be treated seriously. I do not think that those who respond to the suffering by offering to probe, scan, puncture, suction and cut women in repeated experiments are taking that suffering more seriously than I. They are not asking how much of women's suffering has been socially structured and inflicted and is therefore not inevitable. [24]

There are two distinct strands which emerge from this comment. The first relates to attitudes to infertile women and the second to the question of experimentation. The second of these issues I will tackle later, but for the moment, I will concentrate on the former.

What this part of Corea's assertion is saying is that society sets and then systematically reinforces the aspirations of its members in areas such as reproductive decisions, that the agenda is male-dominated and that science and medicine (also male-dominated) then step forward to provide the answers to questions which have already been posed in a biased way. Thus, if the history of society is traced, it can be said to be a history of inequality between the sexes, an inequality which is more than economic and extends to the roles which each gender is **supposed** to play. Patriarchal societies, the argument would continue, have slotted women into specific roles, which cannot fail to influence even current generations. That this is at least in part true cannot be denied. Women make up more than half of the population, yet are often referred to as if they were a minority group. It is a sad comment on a society which claims equality as a goal that **legislation** was needed to attempt to counter overt and hidden discrimination on gender grounds — most of that discrimination being against women.

Outside the sphere of reproduction, of course, women have their gender and biological roles. For example, criminologists, sociologists and others have spent many years concentrating on women's role (and often blaming women for social problems); from criminological theories claiming that women who commit crime are more deviant than their male colleagues, to sociological theories of 'maternal deprivation' as a root cause of social ills. Nor is this concentration on women's reproductive status new. History shows that, 'A woman who failed to produce a child could be reproached, ridiculed and, during the Middle Ages, even burned as a witch'.[25]

Moreover, the shape of the society in which we live is, this argument would continue, dominated by the powerful male who has shaped social institutions to serve himself best. Thus, Robyn Rowland says: 'In the relationship between men and women as social groups, patriarchal values and structures effectively set the limits of women's choice. Social institutions such as the family reinforce and maintain the patriarchal system.'[26]For these feminist theorists, then, the critical impact of social structures which reinforce male standards, is the extent to which women are defined by their contribution to the family (by way of child producing and child rearing) rather than by their other skills and talents. Corea points this out in stark terms:

> The patriarchy filters through all its institutions the propaganda that women are nothing unless they bear a man's children. This message comes at women from every direction. From philosophers, like Arthur Schopenhauer, who

argued in 1851 that 'women exist, on the whole, solely for the propagation of the species'.... From psychiatrists like Dr Bernard Rubin, who asserted that 'Women have a psychobiological drive organisation toward bearing children' .... From priests like Pope Paul VI who declared in 1972 that true women's liberation does not lie in 'formalistic or materialistic equality with the other sex, but in the recognition of that specific thing in the feminine personality — the vocation of a woman to become a mother'.... Century after century, the message seeped deeply into woman. If she cannot produce children, she is not a real woman, for producing children is the function that defines woman.[27]

Into this social phenomenon, then, stepped science, which 'has been viewed as epitomising "manly" characteristics: reason and objectivity'.[28] Women, on the other hand are described by their lack of these characteristics — are said to be emotional and caring. It is worth remembering that the word 'hysteria' is derived from the word for the womb — a reflection, perhaps, of the extent to which women are seen as both emotionally vulnerable and biologically driven. Their biology is also an explanation for all that they are, and permits both definition and medicalisation. As Foucault said in *Madness and Civilisation*, 'the hysterisation of women ... involved a thorough medicalisation of their bodies and their sex'.[29]

Science and medicine share the characteristics of society, and those who manipulate and control them are equally not free of the preconceptions to which this strand of feminist thought would point. As Schmidtke has said, 'Scientists are at least no better and no worse than the society of which they are members'.[30] Two phenomena then, it is argued, spring from this. The first is that to a greater or lesser extent the impetus of science will be towards what satisfies or interests men, or enhances male aspirations.

Given the importance of breeding, men might be thought to have an interest in playing a major role in it, yet it is suggested that — because of biological reality — men are in some way alienated from the 'natural' reproductive process, in that their contribution ends when their sperm is discharged, while the woman's contribution is more lengthy and intimate. Thus, Corea claims, 'When his seed is alienated, man is separated from the continuity of the human species, from a sense of unity with the natural process. He does not actually experience a link between generations.'[31]

Now, although there is considerable medical control over 'natural' reproduction, for example by pressurising women into hospital births, foetal monitoring and so on, residual power still rests with the woman strong enough to challenge the take-over of pregnancy and birth. However, the new technologies offer at least a partial change to this situation. First, because the area of reproductive technology has been dominated by men, the technologies themselves 'are transforming the experience of motherhood and placing it under the control of men. Women's claim to maternity is being loosened; man's claim to paternity strengthened.'[32] Moreover, this argument continues, the technologies level the playing field by 'creating for women the same kind of discontinuous reproductive experience men now have'.[33] Medicalisation, therefore, cannot allow men to breed, but it can disempower those who can do so by reducing their control to a level more equivalent to that of men.

The second phenomenon is that men set the agenda, and hold an increasing amount of power. The end point of this part of the theoretical perspective would be that, 'Reproductive technology is a product of the male reality. The values expressed in the technology — objectification, domination — are typical of male culture. The technology is male-generated and buttresses male power over women.'[34]

In conclusion of this part of the discussion, let me turn briefly to Corea's use of the word 'experiments'. It is not disputed that for medicine and science to progress, research and experimentation are necessary, and that inevitably they will need to test advances, or potential advances, on human subjects. This is a generally accepted aspect of the major breakthroughs made by medicine over the years. However, the radical feminist's understanding of experimentation goes beyond this, and postulates that women — most notably in respect of their reproductive capacities — have been used more frequently, and more damagingly, than others as a vehicle for inadequately tested or researched products, techniques and technologies. The problems resulting from the trials of DES to prevent miscarriage, the difficulties caused by IUDs and so on would be adduced as proof of this.

The question would then be: if medicine in the past has shown scant regard for women, why should we believe that these new technologies will be any different, merely because they are scientifically more sophisticated? As has been said, 'it is as if the "old" reproductive technologies ... and the "new" ones arose out of two separate medical systems, one of which has a clear record of having hurt women, another of which will help women'.[35] And, of course, the medicalisation of reproduction to which I referred earlier, coupled with the male-driven nature of the technologies, also contributes to disempowerment and may even result in women's health being less respected than that of others. As Sherwin says: 'Women are persuaded that only the application of complex technology can meet their needs and therefore they feel compelled to rely on medical authority for their well-being. Doctors have been willing to take extraordinary risks with women's health in the hope of helping them to become mothers.'[36]

And this is not mere rhetoric. Few, if any, of the doctors involved in these technologies to whom I have spoken have been totally sanguine about the extent to which research on the implications and consequences of these technologies has been undertaken. In other words, the risk factors, while many are known, have not yet been as fully explored as they, and many others, might have wished. I will return to this point later.

Whether or not one can wholeheartedly endorse this particular description of our society's current and historical approach to women and their reproductive status, some evidence in its favour comes both from infertile women to whom I have spoken and other informed comment. In the course of making a radio programme I interviewed and listened to a number of women who had been through these modern technologies, successfully or unsuccessfully, or who were contemplating embarking on them. Without fail, their inability to reproduce, even if the problem was their partner's and not their own, was traced to, and firmly rooted in a sense of failure — of themselves and/or their bodies. For some, this may only show that women **are** primarily driven by the urge to reproduce, but for others this is a serious and damaging reflection of the way in which women have been trained to believe in themselves — or not.

In addition, Freely and Pyper note that, 'Women who have had to make difficult fertility decisions often express their feelings by talking about their bodies — how reliable they are, how weak or powerful, who owns them and how they have been treated by others. All this would suggest that fertility means an awful lot more than the ability to have children.'[37]

In other words, and in apparent endorsement of the view described above, some women have come to define themselves as valuable people primarily in terms of the extent to which they have or lack control over their bodies, most clearly and starkly represented by whether or not they can make reproductive decisions. The inability to make such choices reinforces the alleged congruence of womanhood and childbearing, sometimes to the exclusion of other characteristics and capacities. Thus, these women might be said to have absorbed the cultural stereotype attributed to them, viewing themselves as failed human beings — not merely unable to fulfil one function — when certain reproductive choices cannot be made. And this is particularly acute where the choice which cannot be made is one which guarantees social status — as mother and matriarch. The social and psychological impact of this on women, and the wider community, cannot be underestimated. As has been noted: 'one study has found the psychological impact of infertility to be far greater on women than on men. In the study … nearly one third of the women said they felt bad about their bodies and saw themselves as less feminine because of infertility. Only 10 per cent of men reported a negative body image.'[38] A woman who does not believe in herself is a woman restricted in the contribution she can make.

Of course, one obvious response to this might be — in that case, stop whining and give women what they want. Restore their sense of themselves as feminine by making the technology available that permits them to reproduce. For many, however, this is to tackle the wrong end of the problem and to reincorporate into contemporary society the disdain with which infertile women were treated in the past. First, they might say, change the ethos which renders fertility and what it is to be a woman to be so closely merged, and then we may see the beginnings of liberation — the actual capacity of women to make real choices uninfluenced by social caricatures.

The available technologies cannot currently do this. Even although nature's success rate in achieving pregnancy is not particularly high, that of many of the modern technologies is lower still, and the traumas which techniques such as IVF may entail make this relatively low success rate of vital importance in taking an overview of the technologies themselves and the extent to which they ever could give women what they appear to want.

And I say 'appear to want' quite deliberately. If any part of the above is accepted, then it should be clear that the decision to embark on sometimes painful, often unsuccessful and frequently costly treatment is one which is only arguably representative of a free choice. Now, I would readily concede that little that any of us do could, in reality, be said to be totally freely chosen, but where social pressures are so clear the need to create the best possible opportunity for the freest possible decision-making is enhanced.

There are several elements to this. In the first place, we might agree with Corea, that 'Advocates often argue that these technologies do, in fact, bring women new options and choices. But feminists, looking to the background, have pointed out that any discussion of 'rights' and 'choices' assumes a society in which there are no serious differences of power and authority between individuals. Where power differences do prevail, coercion (subtle or otherwise) is apt to prevail.'[39] The fact that significant power imbalances between men and women **do** demonstrably occur in our society is sufficient to cast doubt on the freedom of the choice to access these technologies.

Of course, it is possible to question the freedom of **any** choice by returning to a point I flagged earlier, concerning the information available in making that decision. It is a general rule of law and of morality that for decisions to be of adequate standing they should be predicated on accurate information about risks, benefits and alternatives. Indeed, it is for this reason that medical practice in general is bound by disclosure rules to obtain what is commonly called an 'informed consent'. However, if it **is** the case that research has been limited or inadequate, then this information is not, and cannot be made, available. In the light of this, even if all else were equal, a real choice would be extremely difficult to achieve.

It was this fact, among others, that prompted legislators and others to favour counselling before people enter into any of the reproductive programmes. However, counselling is never non-directive, and perhaps particularly so when its emphasis is on the type of programme most suitable, the risks (as far as they are known) associated with that course of action, and the success/failure rates (again, in as much as they are known). Counselling for remaining infertile is seldom on offer, and yet this remains a choice which for some at least might be the most rational or personally suitable.

Furthermore, society's interests also play a part in determining freedom of choice. In gaining access to reproductive technologies/techniques, women may see themselves as vindicating a right to reproductive freedom, but that so-called right is in fact a chimera. Not only are these technologies often only available to those who can afford them, but other factors play a substantial part in limiting the extent to which we can say that women have rights to make choices.

In the UK, the relevant legislation, while not outlawing access to single women, nonetheless expressly mentions that account should be taken of the 'need' for a father.[40] In other states, such as Western Australia,[41] access is only allowed if the woman is married or has lived in a stable, heterosexual relationship for at least five years. Of course, as many women can testify, the fact of the male's presence at conception is no guarantee of his presence at or after birth, yet this unthinking attempt to reinforce the nuclear family pervades the provision of reproductive services and denies or restricts access to those whose situation is other than conventional. In addition, in the UK abortion is available only on the say-so of the clinicians and not as a right possessed and defined by women,[42] while successive judgments in the United States have effectively limited the so-called privacy right to terminate a pregnancy.[43] As Freely and Pyper put it:

Science and the law may have opened many doors for the infertile and the unhappily pregnant during the past half-century, but that is not the same as saying that people automatically get what they want. Any fertility decision that involves the co-operation of public agencies will be subject to standards set by those agencies, as well as limits dictated by the law.[44]

Moreover, medical and social judgments have been, and continue to be, used to control women's access to programmes[45] and their behaviour throughout pregnancy[46] — the woman becomes an actual or potential foetal vessel, judged by the extent to which she will conform to accepted norms.

So far, I have tried to put reproduction and reproductive choices into a social perspective — to show the extent to which there is a legitimate debate about the assumptions which underlie technological advance and the extent to which there are cultural, social, political and professional pressures and consequences which should be taken account of. I have also attempted to introduce some additional concerns of my own about matters such as the quantity, quality and availability of information which I have suggested would be needed to ensure that choices were as freely made as possible.

There is no doubt that fertility, or its absence, is highly significant for men and women. Whatever the source of the intense desire to have children experienced by many, failure to achieve it can have devastating effects which go beyond the fact of childlessness and can shape a woman's entire self-perception. Freely and Pyper put this rather neatly when they say: 'There is no one more serene, more apparently in control, than the mature adult who has decided not to have children .... There is no one more confused, more stripped of power, than the mature adult who runs into fertility trouble.'[47]

What I have said is not intended to detract from the modern medical miracle, nor to denigrate those who wish to have access to it. Indeed, this kind of argument is:

> not meant to deny that involuntary childlessness is a cause of great unhappiness for many people. Many individuals and couples suffer from their inability to procreate when they choose to do so; many are indeed eager to pursue whatever techniques might be offered to relive this condition. Their motivations cannot be dismissed as irrational or misguided or judged unethical. As long as the technology that offers relief from their condition is available, it is appropriate for individuals to seek access to it.[48]

However, the fact that the technology **is** on offer is a fact which is arguably independent of women's decision-making. Certainly, women will seek access to assisted reproduction when it is available, but this begs the question 'of whether women want these methods of artificial reproduction',[49] a question which, it is suggested, 'will never be put to us, and certainly the decision about whether to go ahead or stop will not be ours so long as society as we know it exists'.[50] In other words, even if the development and use of assisted reproductive technologies can be said to be in part consumer-led, the consumer is equally denied the right to evaluate the benefits and drawbacks and conclude on where the balance rests.

What I have said is a plea for a number of things. First, that women (and their partners, where they exist) are not seduced into believing themselves to be lesser mortals because they cannot reproduce; second, that we all bear in mind the extent to which our perceived problems may be generated by a skewed social structure, and take this into account when putting ourselves at risk;

third, that we also take account of the down-side of these medical advances. It could, for example, be argued as Corea says that, 'they bring new despair. A few years earlier, a woman could at some point, however painfully, come to terms with her infertility, go on with her life, find a way to live it fully. Now there is no easy way off the medical treadmill.'[51] And finally, that we challenge the prevailing view of medicine and science as morally neutral and recognise the extent to which they reflect the inequalities as well as the qualities of the societies within which they function.

For the women to whom I spoke these issues were not in doubt. Many of them described themselves as becoming obsessed with continuing the programme once begun, whatever the costs in personal or financial terms. Others were afraid to embark on treatment for fear of that obsession, and still others were acutely aware that the apparent choice being made available was also a potential trap — if the technology is there, shouldn't they access it rather than come to terms with their situation? They spoke of fractured relationships, of despair and of grieving. Some pointed out that the acceptance of infertility represented one act of grieving, for the children they could never have. Repeated unsuccessful attempts to become pregnant using assisted reproduction brought similar grief, only this time on a monthly basis. Slotting into the role prescribed, perhaps even demanded, by the society in which one lives may seem to be a more simple solution than challenging it, but for some of these women at least, the technologies available to facilitate their adoption of this role were as damaging as the underlying problem itself.

Deciding to use assisted reproductive technologies may seem to be driven by what the individual wants, but this critique would suggest that serious attention should be paid to the extent to which we **can** know that what we seem to want is actually what we **do** want, and how informed our decision to try for it really is.

Moreover, the potential for coercion, for disvaluing and for discrimination is a feature of our not too distant past. The pressures on women may have become more subtle, less overt, more technological but it would be naïve to insist that they have simply and miraculously vanished.

I have neither the right nor the wish to be critical of others' choices, and am also alert to the possibility that my argument may seem to replace one type of devaluation for another. Analysis of this sort must equally be conscious of the subtleties of what it too is saying. It will doubtless come as a relief to many readers that writers like Stanworth whose perspective is centred on the place of women in the reproductive revolution have not been slow to recognise this potential trap.[52] Taken too far, some of what the most radical feminists would argue can be as disvaluing of women as is a philosophy which defines them solely or substantially in terms of their reproductive capacities and choices. In a study of women's psychological approaches to fertility and infertility, for example, Woollett argued that, 'Women's adjustments to infertility are exacerbated by the almost entirely negative view of infertility and infertile women underlying many medical, psychological and feminist analyses. Women find infertility painful and they feel marginalised.'[53]

Without care, this could end up doing much the same thing to women as those arguments which I have sought to challenge. From this perspective, women are classified as victims, unable to make meaningful choices, ignorant of the implications of these decisions, ultimately and inevitably controlled by men. It is well to be aware of this as the other side of the coin. For this reason, amongst others, feminist theories are sometimes shunned by women as well as men. Yet, they do — indeed, I would argue **must** — have a role in informing this important debate. The reproduction revolution has highlighted traditional conflicts and tensions and has also created new ones of its own. In particular, modern technologies have generated the capacity to conceptualise the foetus as an entity separate from the pregnant women, resulting in enforced obstetrical interventions, the attachment of criminal sanctions to those who do not behave 'properly' in the course of their pregnancy[54] and the return of attempts to enforce reproductive practices. This happened recently in the United States, by, for example, offering women a 'choice' between a prison sentence or the implantation of a long-acting (and still experimental) contraceptive device.[55] Women's fertility has long been a political football, and will likely remain so, yet the team playing with it, who chose the playing field and who will carry off the trophies, are not those most directly affected by the outcome of the game. A strong woman's voice is an essential component of relevant discourse.

In particular, my aim is to provide an argument for enhancing the capacity for informed decision-making, not to describe a right or a wrong choice. Feminist critiques should and do seek to do this by providing a different and coherent analysis of what is a highly sensitive and emotive issue. In pointing to what factors may shift our own perceptions of what we are as human beings, and the shape of what we can or should expect of ourselves, feminist critique has much to offer. Where these factors serve to create, or contribute to, a disvaluation of ourselves, they are worthy of serious scrutiny.

In tandem with this, it is important to assess whether or not the tradition of male-dominated medicine and science has contributed to the wresting of power **from** women and **to** the medical establishment. In the process of the professionalisation of medicine, control of reproduction was taken from (female) midwives and handed over to what was then an exclusively male discipline. It should, therefore, be no surprise that the ethos created was one which fitted a particular set of goals, sought to answer a particular set of questions and paid scant attention to interests and aspirations of women. By rendering public what was inherently private, control subtly shifted. The new reproductive techniques consolidate and continue that tradition.

In conclusion, since reproduction is so significant to individuals and their communities — whether the decision is for or against it — when we make choices and develop relevant technologies, we are in part constructing or reinforcing a theory about the individuals who will seek to take advantage of them. It is important that we are aware of the range — the richness and the poverty — of the theoretical perspectives from which we approach what it is to be a woman, a man or just a person who is as free as possible, rather than definable by, and encapsulated within, their biology. In developing perspectives of personhood which are heavily dependent on biology we are constructing a theory of the human being. But as Max Charlesworth has said: 'A theory of human nature should provide some account of the relationship between the "given" biological and physical constraints on human life and the creative element which enables us to elaborate and transform biological dispositions and tendencies and inclinations and give them distinctively human meanings.'[56]

3 Women and Foetuses: Whose Rights?

The capacity of modern medicine to show actual visual images of the human embryo from very early in the pregnancy has raised new and perplexing problems. Once again, the advances in medicine and science have changed the reality of experience — in this case the experience of pregnancy. In many ways, this relatively recent phenomenon is immensely positive. For example, it permits detection of disorders, preparing women and their partners for decisions about whether or not to continue with a pregnancy. Moreover, developments in foetal therapy may permit certain problems to be resolved before birth.

Perhaps inevitably, there is a down side. The perception of the embryo or foetus has also changed. From being a part of the woman's body, it may now be seen as a distinct and identifiable 'individual', as something which is at least the bearer of interests if not of rights. As Harrison has said, 'The foetus has come a long way — from biblical "seed" and mystical "homunculus" to an individual with medical problems that can be diagnosed and treated. Although he cannot make an appointment and seldom ever complains, this patient will at times need a physician.'[1]

The dangers which lurk behind these advances are primarily concerned with the way in which the ability to identify the foetus as a physical entity can impact on the pregnant woman and her rights. Although pregnant women by and large will do everything in their power to ensure that the embryo/foetus which they carry has the best possible environment in which to thrive, modern technologies add subtle pressures to the pregnancy. Identifying the embryo/foetus physically has led inexorably to the attempt to attribute rights to it — rights which, for some, should be vindicated even in the face of objections from the woman. And, of course, photographs of the foetus have proved to be a dramatic and effective tool in the hands of the anti-abortion lobby. The emphasis, therefore, shifts from concern about the woman to concern about the foetus. This shift has profound and far-reaching implications for all women.

Even if we are all agreed that an embryo or foetus should have the best possible start on the path towards birth, and even if we do not wish to discount it as merely a mass of unimportant and morally neutral cells, there are very strong reasons for being concerned about the development of foetal rights. First, if the foetus has rights they can only be vindicated by intrusion on the woman who carries it, and if she is unwilling for that intrusion to take place she may find herself forced none the less to undergo it. Second, there is an inherent fallacy in attempting to find a stage in its development where rights could sensibly or realistically be attributed to what is, for legal purposes, a non-person. As McCullogh and Chervenak point out: 'All accounts about whether or not the foetus possesses independent moral status commit a common error: they seek to find or reject some time, prior to or at delivery, during which the foetus possesses some intrinsic characteristic that in turn generates independent moral status. This matter is endlessly disputed because … it is endlessly disputable.'[2]

In this chapter, I will not repeat this mistake. Although the status to be given to the embryo or foetus of the human species is an important matter, it is almost certainly incapable of resolution by consensus. People's individual or collective morality will relentlessly point them in different directions from each other,

ensuring that agreement is unlikely. As the (UK) Report of the
Committee of Inquiry into Human Fertilisation and Embryology[3]
(Warnock Committee) put it: 'Although the questions of when
life or personhood begin appear to be questions of fact susceptible of straightforward answers, we hold that the answers to such
questions in fact are complex amalgams of factual and moral
judgements.'[4] Like the (UK) *Review of the Guidance on the Research
Use of Foetuses and Foetal Material*[5] (Polkinghorne Report), Warnock
was forced to conclude inconclusively. What each agreed upon,
however, was that the embryo or foetus of the human species was
worthy of **some** respect even if it was not possible to allocate it
a specific place on the moral scale. What we **can** say, then, is that
the human embryo/foetus will always count as more morally relevant than even a fully grown animal, but it will not count as
being as morally relevant as a human child or adult.

Even if it is agreed that this is an appropriate position to adopt,
however, the fact that it has been reached is merely the beginning
and not the end of the problem. Simply to say that some status,
some protection, is the due of the embryo or foetus does not,
manifestly, explain how much. Nor does it tell us when, and in
what circumstances, this moral status is relevant. And this is an
important puzzle, because whatever status we concede to the foetus
is directly relevant to the status which we accord to the woman
who is carrying it. If, for example, we adopt the position that the
foetus is possessed of rights, then there are clear ramifications for
the abortion debate and obvious potential conflicts between the
woman and the foetus. Even if the foetus is only seen as a potential being with interests, there may still be a reason to be concerned
that these interests could be taken as trumping the interests of
others, most notably the pregnant woman.

Although the status to be given to the human embryo/foetus
may seem like an unnecessarily esoteric question, it is one of

increasing practical relevance to women, doctors and the law. The changing face of medicine brings the dilemmas posed into sharper and clearer focus: 'elevation of the foetus to patient status has occurred not because of any change in the foetus or in the maternal–foetal relationship but because of a change in physicians — in how they think about and relate to their patients during pregnancy so it is in the physician–patient relationship that we should expect the ethical repercussions to begin.'[6] Medical technology, for example, permits photographs of early foetuses to be shown, identifying the foetus and giving it credence long before it used to have such to anyone other than the pregnant woman. Control of information concerning the foetus is increasingly clinical. As Wells says:

> Knowledge of the foetus is no longer purveyed from the woman to her doctor, but the other way round. This has paved the way for the development of the movement to protect separately the rights of the foetus. It is no longer perceived in terms solely as part of a woman's body, it has become a site of separate recognition. A movement has developed which seeks to subordinate the pregnant woman to the health and welfare of her foetus.[7]

This movement is often portrayed by the phrase 'maternal/foetal conflict', a term which disguises a number of suppositions and whose very language is designed to sway the listener. First, although the foetus is correctly identified as a foetus, the pregnant woman becomes a 'mother', with all of the implications about caring, protection and so on which that term generally conjures up. Second, the use of the word 'conflict' suggests a battle of sorts, yet there can in fact **be** no conflict since there is only one person — the pregnant woman. Unless the foetus is given a distinct status, there are no adversaries — there is one person, and one potential person. Moreover, the word conflict seems to imply hostilities — and if the implication is that there is hostility, then clearly this can only come from the pregnant woman to her foetus, since the foetus has no capacity to be hostile and cannot deliberately harm the woman who is pregnant. The woman, therefore, must be the person who is hostile — not making decisions in her own best interests, but in hostility to the foetus.

Yet this perception of conflict is one which is insidiously penetrating the consciousness of physicians and their patients. Moreover, its adoption by clinicians has rendered it a matter of legal concern also. The dilemma, therefore, has moved from the arena of morality and has forced the law to address it also. Perhaps because, as Johnsen suggests, the law lacks the framework necessary to conceptualise the debate as anything other than an all or nothing attribution of rights, the foetus is in this model viewed as 'an entity independent from the pregnant woman with interests that are potentially hostile to hers'.[8]

In terms of characterisation of what is going on, these presuppositions are very important. Not only do they subliminally inform the debate but they may, directly or indirectly, predict the outcome. Of course, one very simple approach would be simply to say 'there is no debate' — what we have is one person (who happens to be pregnant) and nobody else. Traditionally this was the legal position. The embryo/foetus has no legal rights. It is not a person until live birth, although rights may be backdated (for example to permit the born child to sue for damage sustained pre-conception or pre-birth, or to inherit under a will). In the recent Scottish case of *Hamilton* v. *Fife Health Board*,[9] a child was born suffering damage which was the result of admittedly negligent treatment before its birth. The child died a few days later and the parents sued for compensation under an Act of Parliament which permitted recovery of damages if a 'person' was harmed by the negligence of another. The question was whether or not the parents of the child could recover on behalf of their son, and the argument against them was that since the child was not a legal person when the harm occurred then he did not qualify as being a 'person' for the purposes of the legislation. In awarding the parents damages, the court accepted that there was no person at the actual time the harm was inflicted, but also said that since the harm only emerged on live birth, then the child was for all intents and purposes a person within the terms of the act at the time the harm actually occurred, because no harm could be caused to a non-person. In other words, the fault and the harm only took on legal significance when the child was born and became a legal person. This view is entirely consistent with maintaining the rights of pregnant women, while at the same time recognising that justice is due to the live-born child, but it does not provoke a conflict nor does it attribute rights to foetuses. What it does do is to endorse the rationale for the development of laws which offer protection to embryos/foetuses (on live birth) without invading the autonomy of women.

But although the laws which allow recovery of damages on live birth for harm which occurred pre-natally or even pre-conception specifically exclude the concept of embryonic or foetal rights, there is no doubt that it would go against the intuitions of some people to suggest that this issue can be dealt with quite so starkly. If we adopt the moral position of Polkinghorne and Warnock, that is that the embryo foetus of the human species is worthy of some respect, then, although we are not looking at two separate, distinct and equal parties, when considering the embryo/foetus we **are** looking at an entity which is deserving of some respect, perhaps implying some special care. And it is this which generates the dilemmas faced by women, doctors and ultimately the law.

First, what is the role of the doctor in relation to the woman and the foetus? Are both of them patients, or is there only one patient, entitled to the best the clinician can offer? This question may prove highly uncomfortable for a doctor, especially if a second consideration is also present — namely that in the view of the doctor something could be done to help the foetus but the woman refuses to agree to it. The frustration of knowing that a foetus could be helped and could be born healthy as opposed to damaged but for the attitude of the woman can readily be understood emotionally, but what happens as a result of this knowledge is dependent on both the moral standing of the foetus and the extent to which women are deemed to have absolute rights to bodily integrity. Robertson and Schulman have noted that:

> Developments in obstetrics, genetics, foetal medicine and infectious diseases will continue to provide knowledge and technologies that will enable many disabled births to be prevented. While most women will welcome this knowledge and gladly act on it, others will not. The ethical, legal, and policy aspects of this situation require a careful balancing of the offspring's welfare and the pregnant woman's interest in liberty and bodily integrity.[10]

In professional terms, therefore, the status of the foetus may be of direct and practical importance. Undoubtedly a doctor owes duties to his/her patient, but this apparently simplistic statement disguises murkier moral questions. A patient is someone with rights. A patient, therefore, must be a person. So, is the foetus a person? Not according to McCullough and Chervenak, who say:

> the foetus cannot be thought to possess subjective interests. Because of the immaturity of its central nervous system, the

foetus has no values and beliefs that form the basis of such interests. It obviously follows from this that the foetus cannot possess deliberative interests, since these, in turn, are based on subjective interests and reflection on subjective interests. The latter is a task no foetus can accomplish. Hence, there can be no autonomy-based obligations to the foetus. Hence, also, there can be no meaningful talk of foetal rights, the foetus's right to life in particular, in the sense that the foetus itself generates rights.[11]

More simply put, the foetus may manifest diagnosable and treatable symptoms which the physician could resolve or palliate, but the patient is the pregnant woman. Only through her can treatment be given and only by her can it be authorised. Nor is the claim that the foetus is not a **patient** defeated by the fact that it could sue after live birth for harm caused by the doctor's negligence while it was still *in utero*. As courts in a number of cases have made clear, the harm only occurs legally on live birth, since no person was present to **be** harmed prior to birth.[12]

Yet despite this apparent legal clarity, it will be seen that this approach is not always the one adopted, with real, sometimes tragic, consequences for the pregnant woman. Despite the lack of agreement on the moral status of the foetus and the legal clarity that the foetus holds no rights, medical advance continues to postulate situations in which the temptation is to override these axioms. As Gregg has said, 'Prenatal technologies can ... influence the relationship between doctors and pregnant patients. Ultrasound, frequently described as a "window on the womb" can promote the medical treatment of two patients: the pregnant woman and her foetus.'[13] Technology can 'make doctors view women and their foetuses as adversaries, instead of assuming that the interests of the mother and her foetus are consistent with one another.'[14] And in a battle of adversaries, one has to 'win'.

Advocates for the rights of women may find themselves defeated by the emotional appeal of arguments in favour of correcting foetal problems. When this situation arises, questions of women's rights may be ignored or side-stepped by clinicians keen to promote health — in other words, the perception of the foetus as a patient triggers the doctor's instinct to heal, even if treatment is uncomfortable, perhaps risky, for the woman. As McCullough and Chervenak have said:

> The viable foetus is not presented to the physician solely as a function of biomedical technology to diagnose, manipulate or treat it — contrary to what seems to be a widespread belief among physicians. This view is mistaken, because it assumes that the pregnant woman is always obligated to accept whatever morbidity and mortality risks are involved for her in obstetric management thought to protect and promote foetal interests.[15]

Yet this is a view which is currently gaining favour. As has been said, 'The earlier model for the woman–foetus relationship was interdependence. Law followed this model. Unborn foetuses had very few legal interests at law. Now, doctors regard the foetus as a separate patient, and the law recognises the foetus as a being with independent interests.'[16] If this is true, and it will be seen later that it seems to be, then pregnant women will see their rights subjugated to these legally recognised interests. The consequences of this are profoundly disturbing. For one thing, it places pregnant women in a uniquely disadvantaged position, by seeming to impose on them a duty to rescue — which would not be imposed under any other circumstances on any other person. As Lew points out, 'It is certain that a court could not order a parent to donate bone marrow in order to save a child's life. Yet courts order pregnant women to submit to surgery for the sake of a foetus. This is illogical, for the born child has constitutional rights, which the foetus does not, and the pregnant woman is subjected to a more dangerous, intrusive procedure than the donor would experience.'[17] Moreover, as Annas has said 'Favoring the foetus [over the mother] radically disvalues the pregnant woman and treats her like an inert incubator, or a culture medium for the foetus.'[18]

It has already been suggested that if we do not concede that the foetus is a person, then we owe it no duties, even if we may offer it some respect. Yet, in a number of jurisdictions, most notably perhaps in the US, that 'respect' seems to have been used as a sword with which to threaten women. Forced obstetrical interventions, aggressively managed pregnancies and so on have resulted in women losing their dignity, rights and even lives — all sacrificed on the altar of foetal protection.[19]

Now, it may be that some, perhaps many, are unconvinced by the argument that the foetus is not a patient because it is not a person. However, even from this perspective, more would be needed by way of argument to justify the overriding of the competently expressed opinion of the pregnant woman. Thus, even if the argument that the foetus is not a patient is unconvincing, McCullough and Chervenak would conclude that, 'the obligation to protect and promote the interests of the patient applies theoretically to all patients equally, even and especially when the physician has more than one patient'.[20] The conclusion of this would, therefore, be that those who would argue that the foetus is a patient could at best only argue that its interests are equivalent in weight to those of women. The doctor would still be obliged to justify choosing one set of interests over the other.

This issue is taken up by Mattingley[21] who analyses the implications of reaching either conclusion as to foetal status. On the one hand, the argument runs, if the pregnant woman and the foetus are seen as one patient, then in calculating risks and benefits of proposed foetal treatment, the doctor must base his/her recommendations on the **totality** of risks and benefits. Mattingley concludes this would mean that, even if there is some risk to the pregnant woman, and some benefit to the foetus, the doctor's conclusion must be a recommendation for therapy.

On the other hand, if the woman and the foetus are seen as separate patients, Mattingley continues, then the doctor's authority to intervene is more restricted since benefit will accrue to one (the foetus) but none will accrue to the other (the woman). In seeking to resolve this problem, doctors will likely turn to the principles of medical ethics for guidance. The modern statement of these comes from Beauchamp and Childress[22] who outline four major principles: beneficence (the obligation to do good), non-maleficence (the obligation to do no harm), autonomy and justice. However, these may not be particularly helpful for the clinician in these circumstances since, with the possible exception of justice, they are individualised concepts and contain within them no capacity or authority to balance the competing interests of patients. The doctor therefore must consider the well-being of each patient as a distinct individual.

Whatever weight we attach to this latter argument — and clearly it may mean that the clinical move towards holding the foetus to be an independent patient actually limits rather than expands the doctor's authority to override the views of a competent woman — as Annas has said, 'Foetuses are not independent persons and cannot be treated without invading the mother's body ....Treating the foetus against the will of the mother degrades and dehumanises the mother and treats her as an inert container.'[23]

But what is the role of the pregnant woman? Does she not have obligations to the foetus which she carries and in whose creation she shared? What kind of woman would set up this potential problem in the first place? As Lew says, 'Conflicts between a woman's needs and those of her foetus are vexing because they pit powerful cultural norms against one another: the ideal of autonomy and the ideal of maternal self-sacrifice.'[24] In any event, could it not be argued that choosing to proceed with a pregnancy rather than terminate it imposes on a woman increased obligations to do whatever is necessary (short of sacrificing her own life) to ensure that the foetus survives and survives in as healthy a condition as possible? If this means some discomfort to her, so be it. Is this not the line we should take?

Simply put, the answer to this is 'no'. As Swartz has said: 'Although it may be morally and ethically appropriate in most cases in which 1) a woman's own health would not be adversely affected and 2) the foetus is viable for the woman to make decisions that would enhance the foetus's chance for good health, legislating for morality in these cases raises more questions than it answers.'[25]

In other words, we may legitimately feel unhappy with the woman who fails to take action which could or would have benefits for the future child and which requires minimal invasion of her bodily integrity, but we should not permit the law to force her to comply with that action. We may not think too much of her, but we should not take the legal power to impose our morality on her. Or as Ruddick and Wilcox put it: 'Perhaps a woman ought to choose abortion or foetal surgery, but it might be wrong to prevent her from choosing the morally impermissible option of a continued, untreated pregnancy.'[26]

Why is this the correct answer? There are a number of good reasons why any attempts to force women into a legal corner concerning their decisions during pregnancy must be avoided. First, the argument from autonomy would support the view that the woman — and only the woman — is a right-bearer in these situations. There is no other (legal) person in existence and nobody else who can consent on the competent woman's behalf. She and she alone is custodian of her physical integrity. As Swartz puts it, 'If pregnant women were treated the same as non-pregnant women and men, their rights to refuse treatment would be relatively clear.'[27]

There is no doubt that individuals have a coherent, morally and legally recognised right to refuse treatment, even where that treatment might save their life.[28] This stems from rights to self-determination or autonomy, and reflects respect for persons. It also protects the desired and desirable voluntariness of the medical enterprise. Thus, for example, courts have refused to force organ donation even when they clearly disapproved morally of the competent refusal, and courts throughout the world have endorsed, with however heavy a heart, the right of individuals to refuse life-saving treatment even when that refusal is irrational or inexplicable in the eyes of third parties.

Yet, when the woman's wishes are subjugated to the assumed interests of the foetus, her right to refuse any and all treatment is placed at risk. In no other situation would one individual's autonomy rights be invaded to protect someone else — even where that 'someone else' is actually alive and a bearer of rights him/herself. A woman cannot be forced to undergo treatment to save the life of her born child, but in some countries she may be forced to do just that in the interests of a non-person. As Purdy says, 'Women, like men, want to control what happens to and in our bodies. Women's ability to do this is being threatened by proponents of the view that our choices should be subordinated to the welfare of foetuses within us.'[29]

That this should be the case is a manifest usurpation by medicine and the law of their positions of trust in the community. It disvalues women and implies the primacy of a being with potential over a being with actuality. As Annas has said, 'The reality … is that the foetus can be treated without its mother's consent only by drastically curtailing her liberty during pregnancy or by subjecting her to major surgery at or near birth.'[30]

A further reason for unease about the law becoming involved in enforcing treatment is that it merely replaces one (arguably) morally dubious decision with a perverse and (unarguably) immoral intrusion into the integrity of a human being. The combination of medical science and the law can be as threatening to liberty in these situations as in the others mentioned in this book. Anecdotal evidence can be unsatisfactory, but one case above all others displays just what I mean.

The US case of Angela Carder[31] shows most starkly the potentially dreadful consequences of losing sight of the respect to which people are entitled. Angela Carder was terminally ill and 26 weeks pregnant. She had indicated that she was willing to accept certain treatment if it meant that she could survive an additional two weeks so as to maximise the chances of her foetus' survival. In the event, her condition deteriorated rapidly, and she required intubation to ease her breathing. The following day, the trial court held a hearing at the hospital following a request from the hospital for a declaratory judgement that a caesarean section could be carried out. At this stage, the foetus was about $26^{1}/2$ weeks' gestation and medical evidence was led which indicated that Mrs Carder's condition was terminal but that there was a chance that the foetus could survive if the surgery went ahead. It was said that it would not be possible to seek her views about the surgery, and in the event no attempt was initially made to ascertain them. In fact, at no stage was she interviewed by the court.

Her family opposed the treatment. Further evidence was subsequently led that Mrs Carder explicitly said (having regained consciousness) that she did not want the surgery, but the court none the less ordered the operation to go ahead. The baby lived for a couple of hours and Mrs Carder for two further days. It requires no imagination to appreciate the devastation wrought to the entire family by this clear and unashamed denial of a dying woman's express wishes. To be sure, lawyers and others may quibble about the condition of Mrs. Carder and her capacity to give or refuse consent, but these are merely speculative attempts to explain away what can only be described as barbarism. So how could a court reach such a conclusion?

The answer, of course, rests on the court's acceptance of two premises which I have argued are erroneous and rights reducing. First, that the foetus (perhaps particularly a viable one) is a separate patient for whom rights or interests can be claimed (this may be especially true of the US situation given its abortion laws which will be considered later in the book). Second, that women's rights can be overridden by the interests of the foetus and can be sacrificed in the event of conflict. Describing this, with considerable restraint as 'far from equitable',[32] Lew makes the telling point that, 'If the law is to treat women as men's equals it must afford women and men the same measure of individual autonomy. Parents who make sacrifices for their children should be encouraged, even lauded, but the law should not require such sacrifices. Self-sacrifice is a gift. Forcing a pregnant woman to sacrifice her health for her foetus is simply slavery.'[33]

For some, this decision is even worse than slavery. Annas describes the decision in this way: 'They [the judges and the doctors] treated a live woman as though she were already dead, forced her to undergo an abortion, and then justified their brutal and unprincipled opinion on the basis that she was almost dead and her foetus's interests in life outweighed any interest she might have in her own life and health.'[34] But the fact that she would inevitably die is (in all situations) a legal irrelevance, although Lew claims, identifying yet a further sinister undertone, that in this case, 'The court was swayed by arguments advanced by the appointed counsel for the foetus and the District of Columbia Corporation Counsel that it should give little weight to Mrs Carder's constitutional rights because she was dying.'[35]

Yet in principle, it is just as much murder to kill someone who would die in the next second as it is to kill someone with 40 years remaining. However, in the purported interests of the foetus, this is precisely what happened here, with the authority of the law, and therefore, until reversed on appeal, with its sanction. In any other situation, this whole scenario would be unthinkable. The first UK case of forced caesarean was decided on the basis of this case[36] — the judge apparently having failed to appreciate that it had been overturned on appeal. Two subsequent cases have reinforced the law's acceptance that foetal interests have considerable weight, although in one case the court ordered surgery on the basis that the woman was not legally competent to refuse it.[37]

However benign the motivation of the doctors, these cases show the rights-stripping potential of this kind of alliance between medical science and the law. It is almost as if the technology is in and of itself the critical issue — we can do it, so we should. The judgement that it should be used is scientific and therefore thought of as rational, explicable and disinterested. When coupled with the emotional appeal of the possibility of rescuing foetal existence, there seems to be an almost unstoppable juggernaut which the pregnant woman is ill-equipped to halt. These cases also point to further reasons why we should not legally seek to enforce particular behaviour on pregnant women. As the Appeal Court in Mrs Carder's case said 'Rather than protecting the health of women and children, court-ordered caesareans erode the element of trust that permits a pregnant woman to communicate to her physician ... all information relevant to her proper diagnosis and treatment.'[38] In addition, the court also noted that the threat of enforced treatment would be likely to drive many women away from seeking pre-natal care in the first place, again putting women and foetuses at potentially increased risk. By the time this case was heard reports suggested that some 36 cases of this sort had been before US courts[39] — a figure which would, if widely known, more than likely result in precisely the consequences which the judges feared.

Yet another strong argument against enforcing specific behaviour in pregnancy is that to do so implies that the woman's decision is somehow flawed. In deciding about her own medical treatment, the woman can be given information and advice but cannot be forced to accept treatment even where it will save her life. The considerations which weigh heavily with her — even if not shared by her doctors or others — must legally be given absolute credence. Yet, where her decision will affect an entity without legal rights, it seems that this fundamental principle flies out of the window. Her reasons are dismissed, discounted or ignored because, on a consequentialist model, we disapprove of the **outcome** of that choice. In other words, in these circumstances the law treats the woman as if she were in the same situation as a child or a mentally disabled person.

The implications of this are either that the woman is of lesser value than the potential of the foetus she carries or that there is an assumption that her reasons are inadequate, perhaps trivial. Yet Angela Carder had been prepared to accept considerable discomfort in an effort to give her foetus a chance. Equally, in less dramatic cases, women should not be assumed to be acting hysterically, selfishly or maliciously when they weigh their own interests against those of the foetus and come down on the side of their own. It is most unlikely that women take such serious decisions lightly and certainly they have little to gain. As Draper says:

in the maternal versus foetal conflict model, whoever wins, pregnant women lose. Resolving the conflict in favour of the mother gives her the liberty and the sole burden for deciding whether or not the foetus will live; she alone must sacrifice or live with the consequences. If the conflict model is resolved in favour of the foetus, women lose out again; since the sacrifice for saving life is extracted from them and them alone.[40]

This has been a necessarily brief account of the dilemmas posed by the apparently conflicting interests of some women and some foetuses. I have tried to show that what is really at issue is the right of women to respect — to the respect that would be shown were they not pregnant or were they of a different gender. Certainly, the fact that there is an embryo or foetus in existence complicates the matter — this is not in dispute. But what is in dispute is why it complicates it and to what extent.

Like most people, I share the view that we should offer some concern to the embryo or foetus, what the Polkinghorne Committee called 'a special status for the living human foetus at every stage of its development which we wish to characterise as a profound respect based on its potential to develop into a fully formed human being'.[41] That it holds no legal status does not necessarily interfere with this desire, although it can and should simplify what can or cannot be done to respect the pregnant woman.

Nor is it antipathetic to argue that the decision on intervention is solely and exclusively for the pregnant woman. Respect is desirable, but can be overridden where other interests predominate, as they should in this situation. Nor is this an unusual conclusion. We hold certain rights to be inalienable, such as the right to life, but we equally concede that in certain circumstances life may be taken. These circumstances generally arise where the

effect of not taking the life would be worse than the taking of it.
If this is the case where fundamental human rights are concerned,
then surely it provides a strong reason for viewing the pregnant
woman and the foetus in the same way. In other words, the effect
of dealing with the woman in such a way that her human rights
are ignored is a greater harm than the good of treating the foetus
(who is not a person).

Moreover, accepting that foetuses have rights has had consequences beyond forced obstetrical interventions. In some countries
the criminal law has been utilised to punish women for behaviour during their pregnancy. Ikenotos records these incidents,
noting that 'The criminal prosecution of women for acts against
foetuses is the strongest form of reinforcing the ideology. The
message that bad mothers should be punished is expressed when
criminal law is utilised.'[42] Although civil litigation following pre-
natal harm and a live birth is permitted, we do not routinely see
pharmaceutical companies being prosecuted, say for distributing
drugs with teratogenic effects, yet women may be prosecuted for
behaviour which is objectively no worse, and which may even have
occurred at a time when they were unaware of being pregnant.
The logic of this would lead to the conclusion that — to avoid
criminal (and civil) liability — all fertile, sexually active women
of childbearing age should act at all times as if they were pregnant. Such constraints on the freedom to live life as we choose
would certainly never be accepted in any other situation.

Nor is it merely in the criminal law that biology has been used
to limit women's full participation in the community. Bayer[43] notes
a report in the *New York Times* on 4 January 1979 that a number of
female employees had opted for sterilisation as the only way to
keep their current jobs. The company concerned had indicated
that since certain jobs exposed women to substances which might
harm foetuses, and since this risk could not be eliminated, the

women would be moved to different, poorer paid positions. This is an even further step, since the company was purporting to act in the interests of **potential** foetuses.

Despite the gross invasion of liberty represented by these practices, the law continues to endorse the purported interests of the foetus and the clinical recommendation for intervention. It does this by dint of adopting three interlinked rationales. First, the state has an interest in foetal welfare — an interest which may increase with the gestational age of the foetus. Second, that the clinical recommendation is effectively value free, in that — presumably unlike the woman's decision — it is rational and scientific. This reinforces my theme: that disvaluing of choice and restriction on vindicating rights can result from handing authority over the moral content of actions to medicine and science. The result, it is claimed, is an apparently inevitable transformation of the law from a system designed to uphold certain values to a structure with limited, and professionally dominated, tests at its disposal. As Ikenotos says, 'The result is that widely disparate human situations are treated as problems in conformity.'[44] Moreover, this conclusion also reinforces the argument that there is a therapeutic or scientific imperative which is given undue weight. Ikenotos continues, 'We default to science when we assume that if the technology is there, we should use it, and then we act on this assumption without critical evaluation of the wisdom of acting.'[45]

Third, the capacity of science to present the embryo or foetus to us in visual form, leads to the conceptualisation of the foetus as a patient — as a right or interest bearer. The doctor, therefore, acquires duties to treat, even if that treatment necessarily invades the woman's rights. Yet, 'History shows that intervention often occurs for the sake of intervention and…with no specific evidence of necessity. The increase in intervention has consistently been explained by referring to foetal interests.'[46]

With its customary deference to medicine and science, the law appears sanguine about reinforcing biological stereotyping, donning the mantle of the arbiter of clinical/scientific enquiry rather than that of the upholder of rights. Failing to address matters like this as human rights issues forces complex dilemmas into a framework which permits of professional rather than humane enquiry and resolution. Yet again, the law is happy to hand over authority to the physicians, apparently heedless of the personal and social cost associated with such derogation of responsibility. In weighting the scales so heavily in favour of clinical recommendation, based on capacity rather than morality, it 'treats women as wombs as a matter of law'.[47] Additionally, as Cook and Plata wrote, 'Laws and policies stereotype, confine and punish women because of their role in reproduction.'[48]

We may all desire that every pregnant woman act in an unimpeachable manner — many, if not most, do — but we cannot enforce this. To seek to do so would entail an unwarranted intrusion into all aspects of a woman's life solely because of the fact of her pregnancy. It would logically entail that the clinical information we have (not all of it unarguable) concerning what has the potential to harm the foetus would become not information or advice but an authoritarian regimen, removing freedom of choice for the duration of the pregnancy. It engenders, or perpetuates, discrimination against women based on their biological capacities — a form of discrimination which is certainly outlawed in the United States. As Johnsen says, 'by regulating women as if their lives were defined solely by their reproductive capacity, the state perpetuates a system of sex discrimination that is based on the biological differences between the sexes, thus depriving women of their constitutional right to equal protection of the laws'.[49] This right should be equally respected in countries with no written constitution.

Showing respect for the embryo/foetus at the expense of women's rights is a monumental misunderstanding of the concept of respect and a perverse interpretation of the value of human rights. It is to the law's shame that it has in the past colluded in this to the detriment of women.

4 A Woman's Right to Choose?
Law, Medicine and Abortion

The abortion debate has undoubtedly become one of the most divisive and bitter of the last few centuries. Dworkin says, 'Abortion is tearing America apart. It is also distorting its politics, and confounding its constitutional law.'[1] Although the debate in other countries is less fierce, abortion remains a political and social 'hot potato'. As an issue, it is both distinct from and yet allied to the tensions between the rights of pregnant women and the interests of embryos and foetuses. Although this debate does not have its roots in technology, and the arguments are based on historical as well as modern ideologies, it shares some characteristics with the arguments discussed in the previous chapter.

It is commonly assumed that the twentieth century has seen the liberalisation of abortion laws which previously had been strict and uncompromising. A brief look at the history of abortion law and practice will show just how erroneous such a belief is, and analysis of current law will highlight the extent to which the slogan 'A woman's right to choose' is not yet fully vindicated.

It is acutely poignant that the current control over women's choice in this area is not based on any immutable truth, but is rather the product of social, professional and religious pressures, given the force of law, which can by no means be said to have been consistent over the centuries. Just as religions modified and developed their notions about the time of ensoulment (and therefore moral value), so societies have changed their views on abortion. Some early societies, for example, seem to have found little difficulty in countenancing pregnancy termination. On the other hand, the basis of Western medical ethics — the Hippocratic oath — has been used mantra-like to dictate the ethics of the profession of medicine as it emerged in the nineteenth century, and has proved a convenient tool for the prohibitions on abortion which emerged most significantly at that period of history. Further, the combination of medicalisation with the customary legal deference to scientific and medical development has altered the nature of the debate in a way which requires considerable sophistication from those who seek to address the full complexity of women's demands. A brief look at of the history of abortion will show that there is nothing inevitable or fixed about social and other attitudes to it.

Until its latter stages, the Roman Empire is often regarded as the apotheosis of civilisation. Its restrictions were at least matched by its liberality. As Luker points out, in that society 'abortion was so frequent and widespread that it was remarked upon by a number of authors. Ovid, Juvenal and Seneca all noted the existence of abortion, and the natural historian Pliny listed prescriptions for drugs that would accomplish it. Legal regulation of abortion in the Roman Empire ... was virtually non-existent.'[2] This, of course, does not mean that there were no controls over its practice, but rather that there was little law in its respect even in a society which prided itself on its legal framework — a model for a number of jurisdictions even today. Potentially, of course, abortion was controlled in other ways, for example by the ethical codes of the emerging artisans who would become the modern-day physicians. Certainly, there is a widespread presumption that — at least for those who belonged to the school of Hippocrates — the oath to which they swore allegiance would preclude involvement in the termination of any pregnancy.

However, it must be remembered that, despite the extent to

which the modern physician may rely on the Hippocratic Oath as a basis for his/her practice, it is a strange hybrid, and its interpretation and use are at best inconsistent and at worst disingenuous.[3] What is clear is that the oath was as much a 'closed shop' agreement as it was a code of ethics. In other words, much of its content is not a statement about the ethical conduct of medicine in relation to patients, but is rather a collection of professional obligations to colleagues, much in the same way as people swear allegiance to schools and countries. Even more interestingly, those parts of the oath which do relate to the physician–patient relationship are as much honoured in the breach as in the observance. Prohibitions on surgery, charging for services and the commitment to the provision of free education in some circumstances are routinely ignored. Indeed, given that the tradition of taking the oath on graduation has largely died away, it is arguable that many doctors do not even realise that these elements are contained in the Oath. Modern statements of medical ethics, whilst more relevant to contemporary medical practice, nonetheless claim the Oath as their source, whilst — perhaps paradoxically — being extremely selective about which parts of the oath they have chosen to hold on to.

But other influences were also at work. In the Christian era some regulation of pregnancy termination by law did exist, although Luker suggests that it 'was designed primarily to protect the rights of fathers rather than the rights of embryos'.[4] Historically, this would be entirely plausible as an explanation. The importance of lineage, and therefore the significance of the father's interest in having offspring (particularly, of course, male offspring) has remained a part of our culture even today. Any argument, therefore, would be unlikely to be couched in terms of a conflict of rights. The male was the only right-holder within this conceptual framework and neither women nor embryos/foetuses would have any standing as even the most feeble competitor.

Of course, grandiose statements of 'ethics' may in any event have little impact on the 'real' world. Whatever the theoretical position, women continued to have unwanted or dangerous pregnancies and to seek ways of avoiding the emotional and/or physical consequences of this. The lack of effective contraception meant that abortion or abstinence were really the only options. The latter, of course, was not so much an option as a punishment. Women's social and economic status was entirely linked to marital and parental status — an attitude enforced by social and legal mores.

Yet, perhaps in the absence of organised opposition, at the beginning of the nineteenth century, the law in many countries, such as the United States, contained no statutory control over abortion. By the beginning of the next century, however, the picture was very different. There are probably several reasons for this. One major contributory factor may well have been the coming together of women as what has been called 'a self-conscious interest group that claimed abortion as a right'.[5] This must have had an impact, in particular since women were also banding together to argue for the more general right to control the number and spacing of their pregnancies. Just as with the organised campaign in twentieth-century Britain for the enfranchisement of women provoked an intense — sometimes vitriolic — backlash, so too it seems plausible that the emergence of the early women's movement would have resulted in an equally organised opposition.

But there was one further, and probably more important, social and political change occurring simultaneously — the drive for professionalisation in the field of medical. The distinguished commentator, James Mohr,[6] puts it succinctly. As he says 'The anti-abortion crusade became at least in part a manifestation of the fact that many physicians wanted to promote, indeed to force where necessary, a sense of professionalism, as they defined it, upon their own colleagues'.[7] It is a recognised characteristic of professionalism that the aspiring profession gathers to itself the monopoly of certain discrete areas of competence and expertise. The relatively unregulated situation in respect of abortion, often seen as a conspiracy of women helping each other, was a threat to the emerging profession of the physician.

Two powerful influences were therefore at work. First, the increasingly assertive demands of at least some women for (albeit limited) reproductive control, and second, the organisation and increasingly scientifically credible practice of medicine. But there was also, as there is today, a symbiosis between the latter and the law. Doubtless, legislators were influenced by the demands and claims of their respected professional colleagues, and the latter part of the nineteenth century saw the emergence of legal controls over pregnancy termination, for example in the Offences Against the Person Act of 1861 (England and Wales). At about the same time, some religions began to identify a clear moral status to be attributed to the embryo or foetus, signalling the beginning of the serious confrontation between foetal and female interests.

The combination of morality, medicine and the law also provided fuel for the professionalisation process and for the removal of abortion control from (female) friends, relatives or midwives. The emerging medical profession was not slow to capitalise on this fortunate congruence of the social and the scientific. On the moral front, women were seen as committing a sin in relieving themselves of pregnancies — the product of conception was morally relevant and women required, in the best traditions of paternalism, to be protected from sinning. Further, elementary scientific knowledge claimed to be able to prove that the embryo was a person from the moment of conception, an assertion for science which nowadays would be regarded with polite scepticism were it to be made.

Moreover, the changes beginning to occur in the law in a number of countries, while possibly **generated** (at least in part) by medicine's claims, also provided a **vindication** for them. As McLaren says, 'The fact that abortion was illegal was taken as reason enough for the medical profession to support the notion that it was both medically and morally wrong; it would only condone the termination of a pregnancy by a surgeon if a mother's life was in danger and full medical consultation took place.'[8]

According to Petersen:

By the beginning of the twentieth century, the medical profession was an increasingly powerful body which was in the process of consolidating its professional status. It held a prominent position in the community and was actively involved in legal and social developments. As the welfare of citizens became a more significant issue, the profession assumed jurisdiction over an increasingly wide range of human affairs. Medicine began to compete with, and gradually displace, the authority of religious institutions and the law.[9]

The medicalisation of women's reproductive choice was effectively complete.

What had been (and remains) an essentially female experience became conceptualised as an inherent part of the male world and subject to male control. The male orientation of the medical world imposed, however innocently, its own values and standards on reproductive choice. As Jackson, et al. say, 'The establishment of modern science and medicine created a male monopoly over what had once been a woman's own sphere of influence: pregnancy and childbirth. These processes have been medicalised, defined as illnesses, and subject to increasing technological intervention.'[10]

The extent of the law's endorsement of the claims made by medicine, and the alacrity with which they were adopted, led to extremely restrictive abortion laws — laws which paradoxically then came under attack from the profession which had been so instrumental in their creation. Having won the technical fight, the differences of opinion between physicians were set to emerge and would serve to reopen and reshape the debate yet again. Some authors, in fact, doubt that there ever was truly a general agreement as to the morality of abortion among doctors. By implication, if this is so (and it seems more plausible than not) the law was reacting to an inherently cynical exercise — the sacrifice of women's control over their lives for the 'greater good' of the recognition of doctors as professionals.

But there was even more to it than this. The tightening of the laws on abortion led to a demand for illegal terminations, since neither doctors nor the law could stop the incidence of unwanted pregnancies. The illegality of abortion created a group of untrained and sometimes unskilled abortionists. Women's lives were on the line in their search for the freedom of choice which they increasingly claimed as a right. Doctors, therefore, ended up by arguing for the liberalisation of abortion laws, at least in as much as this would serve to preserve the lives of these women.

Preservation of female life eventually became an acceptable basis for the relaxation of abortion laws — but since this was a matter in which doctors could claim a discrete competence, the clinician played a vital and central role. Luker, for example, suggests that one principal rationale for medical control of pregnancy termination was its intimate connection with health. Yet advances, particularly in pre-natal and obstetrical care, meant that the threat to women's health posed by pregnancy and abortion was significantly reduced. As she puts it, 'As "preserving the life of the woman" in the physical sense of the word became a medical rarity, the continuum [of the argument for medical control of abortion] collapsed and the consensus broke down. For the first time since the nineteenth century, medical technology … set the stage for abortion to re-emerge as a political and moral issue.'[11] The requirement of physical (and therefore regular medical) evidence was further eroded by the 1939 English case of *R* v. *Bourne*.[12] In this case, the young woman on whom the termination was carried out had been the subject of an horrific rape. Although physically fit, her mental health was felt by the doctor to be in doubt if she were forced to continue with the pregnancy. He therefore carried out the termination and notified the authorities accordingly. The court accepted that he had not breached the current law by extending the definition of preservation of life to cover mental as well as physical health — a major step forward for women, even although it is not possible to predict what would have been the decision had the circumstances of the case been less dreadful.

At the same time, society was changing dramatically. The effects of world war, economic uncertainty and the emergence of powerful political innovation had their own impact on the politics of sex, sexuality and reproduction. In an authoritative work, Rowbotham[13] notes that the social revolution of the twenties and thirties had a profound impact (at least in parts of Europe) on attitudes towards sexual matters. As she says, 'the prevailing dogmatic orthodoxy dismissed sexual and personal questions and ignored the political significance of the manner in which human beings experienced and expressed their lives in sexual relations. Because sexual pleasure was seen as a diversion, which had to be tolerated in moderation because of some of the comrades' weaknesses, it was easy to dismiss the demand for control over the reproduction of self through sexuality as well as through economic production.'[14]

Stripped of certainties, faced with major social, political and economic challenges and with no further overwhelming need to follow a monolithic pursuit of status, cracks began to appear in the facade of cohesion which had once characterised the medical approach to pregnancy termination. As Luker says 'Once there came to be an obvious difference of opinion among physicians about the moral status of abortion rather than the technical grounds for it, the control of abortion was open to new claims.'[15]

By the late 1930s, however, although some countries had liberalised abortion laws almost completely, the majority still retained fairly restrictive positions. Given that the medical profession was unlikely to give up its control over pregnancy termination (among other reproductive issues) and in view of the fact that clinical input undoubtedly rendered abortions safer, a new drive to protect women's health began to predominate in the debate. The discovery of safer abortifacient techniques, coupled with the availability of the means to control infective agents made regulated abortion a more attractive proposition than the continued toll of illegal abortion on women's lives. However, the control of both of these developments was restricted to the medical profession by laws which precluded terminations in general and placed the capacity to acquire and dispense certain products firmly in the hands of doctors.

Social and political change also encouraged the use of the language of human rights in this, as in other, areas. Just as with the 'conflict' between pregnant women and foetuses, a central tenet is concerned with the attribution of rights. Into the arena stepped two polarised views, however, of who actually had these rights. For the anti-abortion lobby, it is the rights of the foetus which predominate, for the pro-choice adherent, the woman's rights are always paramount. To the extent that both opponents and proponents of abortion use the same language, but imply very different things by it, the debate seems likely to be unresolved and may be unresolvable.

In common with the rest of the topics covered in this book, this fundamental difficulty is exacerbated by the extent to which medicine and science are permitted by law to play a key, if not determinant role, in the interpretation of human rights and their vindication in law. As Petersen points out, 'The medicalisation of abortion and the ideology of professionalism have resulted in the medical profession and individual medical practitioners having a considerable influence over the shaping of abortion laws .... The attitudes of referring doctors are ... also important because they perform a gatekeeping function.'[16]

The professional and moral commitments of doctors have undoubtedly influenced the argument surrounding pregnancy termination and have helped to shape both law and social practice. The effect of this has been to widen further the gap between the adversaries in the debate. Moreover, even in countries where the arguments over termination have been less violent than, say, the United States, the emerging science of pre-implantation and pre-natal screening seems likely to add a further dimension to the debate — one which, yet again, is firmly rooted in medical capacities.

The ability to control reproduction is a central and unshakeable tenet of the advocates of women's rights. As Wikler has said, 'The notion of "choice" has served as an ideological cornerstone of the political programme of the movements for reproductive rights and women's health. Feminists have been unequivocally "pro-choice" in their support of a woman's right to choose abortion and contraception over pregnancy'.[17] As will be seen later, this 'choice' is not unlimited, nor is it simply about pregnancy, childbirth and parenting. Nor is it about devaluing the developing embryo or foetus. Rather it has far-reaching consequences for the status of women as equal partners in society — a society which both needs and should value women's engagement with it. Gaining control of reproductive liberty is not a desire based on callousness or indifference towards the embryo/foetus, nor does it necessarily imply that those fighting for it entirely dismiss the embryo/foetus. As Dworkin says:

> It is true that many women's attitudes toward abortion are affected by a contradictory sense of both identification with and oppression by their pregnancies, and that the sexual, economic, and social subordination of women contributes to that undermining sense of oppression. In a better society, which supported child rearing as enthusiastically as it discourages abortion, the status of a foetus probably would change, because women's sense of pregnancy and motherhood as creative would be more genuine and less compromised, and the inherent value of their own lives less threatened.[18]

This is not to say that women would not still seek to terminate pregnancies, but it seems to indicate that when the arguments are couched solely in terms of bodily control, without analysis of the additional reasons which women legitimately have for seeking such control, or the debate focuses on foetal 'rights', then a key component of the relevant issues is missed. Over the years pro-choice writers have rendered their arguments more sophisticated with precisely this point in mind. However, the dominant perception of abortion decisions remains disappointingly uninformed by this discourse and unhappily reinforced by third party assumptions about women's interests, motivations and attitudes which mirror the traditional paternalistic stance of medicine, and through medicine, of the law. As Jackson, et al. say 'Women by no means always concur with medical definitions of their reality, but the privileged status accorded to medical knowledge and the institutionalised power of the medical profession often undermine alternative versions of women's experience.'[19]

In some countries, for example, the United Kingdom, therefore, the abortion debate — while reopened and heading for some liberalisation of the law — nonetheless remained constrained by medical input. The Abortion Act of 1967 — which was a relatively early relaxation of statutory regulation of abortion — was explicitly designed to tackle the question of the high incidence of maternal death following 'back-street' abortions. It neither did, nor intended to, give rights to women. Rather, it relied (as the current UK regulations still do) on the clinical assessment of entitlement to pregnancy termination. But, in line with the decision in *R* v. *Bourne,* it recognised a range of circumstances in which — with medical permission — pregnancies could lawfully be terminated. Subsequent amendment to the 1967 Act has broadened the law in ways which will be considered later.

The British situation can be legitimately criticised on two major counts. The first is that it offered no rights — it was set against a practical rather than a rights-based framework. Second, it continued the tradition of assuming the medical monopoly on gatekeeping — on the provision of authority which triggered the capacity to fulfil the woman's decision. In that respect, it continues (however it is interpreted in practice) to reinforce both the medical model and the tradition of legal deference to perceived clinical superiority.

Several years after the UK legislation, in the United States case of *Roe* v. *Wade*,[20] yet a further step appeared to have been taken. In this case, the US Supreme Court appeared to concur with the perception of the issue as being one primarily of women's rights, rather than the somewhat uncomfortable compromise reached in the United Kingdom. Set against the

Constitutional provision of rights, the Supreme Court apparently addressed women as individuals with specific claims (in this case built around the construction of a 'privacy right') whose satisfaction was to be guaranteed by the law, subject to the limitations which are generally accepted to circumscribe any human or constitutional right.

In this case, the Supreme Court enunciated a set of criteria on which the abortion decision could be based. In developing the so-called trimester system, the Court concluded that in the first three months of pregnancy, the woman had an absolute right to terminate her pregnancy, in the second three months, the state could impose conditions which reflect its interest in both the woman and the developing foetus. In the third trimester (roughly equivalent to what was then thought of as the time of viability), the state has a compelling interest in regulating abortions.

Although hailed as a landmark (which in many ways it was) *Roe* v. *Wade* nonetheless did not entirely — despite its human rights rhetoric — divorce itself from the medical model. Even during the first trimester, when allegedly the woman is given the right to make her own decision, the Court specifically said that 'the abortion decision and its effectuation must be left to the medical judgement of the pregnant woman's attending physician'.[21] The constraints on women's freedom to choose termination which could be imposed after the first trimester were also in large part health related — either resulting from the clinically assessed state of foetal development or through the inevitable constraints on health care budgets — a particular problem in the United States. A number of subsequent cases, whilst claiming not to repeal the Roe approach, have shown just how easily these health related considerations can be used effectively to limit access to pregnancy termination whilst at the same time maintaining the rhetoric of human rights.[22]

Significantly, of course, the trimester framework carried within it the seeds of its own destruction. Or as Justice O'Connor put it, it was 'on a collision course with itself'.[23] By importing the medical into an allegedly human rights based construct, the scheme opened itself to obsolescence. As medical capacity to salvage foetal existence progressed, as it foreseeably would, the rigid enforcement of an outmoded concept of the time at which viability was reached would likely become less and less tenable (as in fact was the experience under the Infant Life Preservation Act of 1929 in England and Wales). Despite the lessons which could be learned from this, it is worthy of note that debate surrounding the Human Fertilisation and Embryology Act of 1990 (UK) concentrated much more intently on the setting of an upper age limit for abortion (which was informed by the medical assessment of viability) than it did on any other issue. Of course, this is entirely in line with the UK approach to abortion, but it nonetheless demonstrates the extent to which even an apparently fragmented medical profession can, both historically and contemporaneously, influence such an important area.

The position in both jurisdictions, therefore, is that the law has been informed, defined and controlled by medical information about the foetus. In line with the arguments in the previous chapter, this has had profound consequences on what pregnancy termination means to women and their rights to make choices about their own bodies. As I said earlier, the liberty to decide may or may not in fact result in a truly free choice, but it is certain that a free choice will never be possible unless reproductive liberty (including the right to terminate pregnancies) is seen as an issue which transcends clinical 'facts' and medical capacities and becomes focused on the real issue — namely, women's freedom from the biological lottery.

Of course, access to contraception and sterilisation have gone some way towards rendering this more feasible, but it would be naïve to suggest that abortion will ever cease to be an issue. The picture, then, has evolved. From being framed by the interests of the medical profession in taking to itself a discrete body of knowledge and competence, the landscape has been further complicated by postulating conflict between the participants — namely the woman (who must protect and fight for herself) and the embryo/foetus, which is protected by doctors and the state.

In a fascinating analysis, Ginsburg suggests that the furore over the judgement in *Roe* v. *Wade* might have been more muted had the abortion question been viewed as one of sexual equality rather than as one which, in her words, left 'the woman tied to her physician'.[24] Recognising reproductive autonomy as an issue far broader than foetal and maternal interests, she points out that, 'the shape of the law on gender-based classification and reproductive autonomy indicates and influences the opportunity women will have to participate as men's full partners in the nation's social, political, and economic life'.[25] Indeed, were it not for the credibility given to the lobby which claims that foetuses have 'rights', and were the issues looked at in the abstract, any state which deliberately chained more than 50 per cent of its talented and productive citizens to biological shackles would be regarded as bizarre.

As Ginsburg continues, 'The conflict … is not simply one between a foetus's interests and a woman's interests, narrowly conceived, nor is the overriding issue state versus private control of a woman's body for a span of nine months. Also in the balance is woman's autonomous charge of her full life's course … her ability to stand in relation to man, society, and the state as an independent, self-sustaining, equal citizen.'[26] Acknowledgement of this as the central issue would, she insists, have meant seeing 'the public assistance cases as instances in which, borrowing a phrase from Justice Stevens, the sovereign had violated its "duty to govern impartially"'.[27]

But the debate is now set to move one step further. The apparent liberalisation of abortion laws was also in part **informed** by clinical input. So too, unless we reassess our approach, will be the abortion practice of the future. Advances in medicine now permit pre-implantation and pre-natal diagnosis, even foetal therapy. Already these capacities have had an impact on the abortion decision. Wikler notes, for example, that 'Recently enacted legislation [in the US], for instance, requires women to undergo the expense and risk of ultrasound tests, presumably to ascertain gestational age.'[28] As was seen in the previous chapter, medicine now has immense potential for diagnosis pre-birth, but this does not simply create an apparent conflict between a woman and her foetus, it also affects the nature of the 'choice' which a woman makes.

Undoubtedly, most women (and their partners) want to give birth to a healthy child. The availability of techniques which can ostensibly achieve this will be, and indeed are already, immensely appealing to the intending parent. In fact, of course, we are already well used to the application of pre-natal screening techniques such as Chorionic Villus Sampling or amniocentesis. The logical outcome of screening programmes is admittedly the termination of an affected pregnancy. No matter one's attitudes to abortion, the earlier such screening can be carried out, the less morally relevant and the less problematic may seem the selecting out of those who are genetically 'deficient'.

Although it may be true that people want healthy children, the drive to find ways of detecting those who will not be has been dominated by medicine. Most recently, this is true of the so-called 'genetic revolution' which allows certain conditions to be located on certain genes.[29] Advances in parallel with this genetic enquiry combine to provide more apparent choice. As Petersen points out, 'In the broad global sense, it is becoming more apparent that debate on abortion cannot be isolated from technological advances. Developments in assisted reproduction and foetal technology have added a new dimension to the issue.'[30]

Luker puts the issue even more starkly: 'given the history of abortion in America [and elsewhere], none of us should be too surprised if, by the turn of the century, technological changes were once again to make abortion a battleground for competing social, ethical and symbolic values'.[31] In fact, this is already happening, driven by the juggernaut of medical advance. It is as if the mere involvement of the clinical somehow changes the nature of the event.

This has two clear consequences. First, it means that decisions may be taken about the embryo or foetus which we would never dream of making about a born child. This is not an argument against permitting women to make such decisions, but rather highlights the double standards which prevail when technology proceeds as if it had no down-side. More worryingly, it places an additional constraint on women's decisions about whether or not parenting is what they seek. Second, it has an impact on choice.

To take the first point, even those who most loudly oppose abortion are much more ambivalent about terminations which are the result of diagnosed foetal handicap. As Rothman notes, 'These abortions, abortions to prevent the birth of a disabled child, are among the most socially acceptable of abortions. In the United States, over 80 per cent of people approve of the use of abortion in this situation.'[32] In the UK, thanks to recent legislation, termination on the grounds of severe handicap is permitted up to full term of the pregnancy.[33] The only other situation where this is possible is the probably uncontroversial exception where termination is necessary to save the woman's life.

Moreover, those who are undergoing assisted reproduction or who fear that they may transmit a deleterious gene may now have available to them the possibility of pre-implantation diagnosis. Furedi, in fact, says, 'In years to come, hopefully within the next decade, it may be as widely available for those with genetic problems as IVF is for infertile couples today.'[34] Yet, she also acknowledges that of the diagnosis in those cases which had already occurred in the UK, in about 7 per cent of the pregnancies the diagnosis was wrong.[35] Two things follow this. First, are we really finding ourselves in a situation where we might actually find the **encouragement** of pregnancy terminations, even given that the diagnosis may result in the discarding of a healthy embryo? And second, the question must be asked, for what are we testing? The assumption that genetic diagnosis is invariably accurate is one which simply cannot be made. Hubbard and Wald point out that:

> Most pre-natal tests offer little precise information. They can suggest problems, but cannot say how significant these problems may be. Genetic predictions, like all medical tests, involve setting arbitrary norms. People, or foetuses, who fall outside them are by definition 'abnormal', irrespective of whether they exhibit noticeable symptoms or whether these symptoms are particularly debilitating. Women are aborting foetuses because physicians have diagnosed a chromosomal irregularity, even though no one can say whether this irregularity would have noticeable effects. Those who refuse to accept such definitions often face reactions ranging from disbelief to hostility.[36]

As more and more conditions receive the clinical label of being genetically determined, are we sure that the questions we are asking are relevant? Claims to have found the gene for delinquency, alcoholism, homosexuality and so on suggest that we are merely a collection of pre-determined characteristics. Any characteristic which is thought of as being undesirable might then logically become the subject of exclusion from the gene pool by means of abortion. Yet, who decides what is undesirable? Manifestly, if the present clinical dominance in decision-making continues, this will be in very large part the scientists and the doctors who asked the question in the first place. Women may not care about, for example, the sexual orientation of their offspring, but we can be fairly sure that — once it is possible to find it out — pressure will be there (because of the attitudes, for example, of others to the gay man or lesbian woman) to decide that a life spent with that particular stigma may not be one worth living. And, as was said earlier, it may be easier for society to condone — even facilitate — terminations where the 'bad' gene can be identified early in the pregnancy, or in the case of pre-implantation diagnosis, before the pregnancy has even been established. Questions about genetic screening will be considered later in the book, but for the moment it is worth pointing to the influence genetic information can have at even this early stage.

This is reminiscent of the problems discussed in the previous chapter and also leads to the second major consequence of medical advance — namely the impact on choice. Whether done pre-implantation or pre-natally, there is, as has been said, a presumption that women will 'choose' not to continue with an affected pregnancy. But, as Hubbard and Wald say, 'The mind-set behind genetic testing rests on societal views of disabilities that should not go unchallenged.'[37] But women are part of society, and a society which tells them that the opportunity is there to avoid births which will be emotionally and financially costly, may also influence their capacity to make a free decision. Pressure to abort —

even given scientific uncertainties — may increase as more and more 'problems' are traced to identifiable clinical conditions.

Yet again, therefore, medicine will have a profound impact on women's lives — perhaps rather poignantly by reversing the process away from making abortion difficult to making it almost expected. The repeated handing over to doctors of the role of moral gatekeeper also imposes more on women. The doctor can see him or herself as merely providing value neutral information, even when coupled with advice, but the responsibility is ultimately borne by the woman, seduced by clinical expertise but abandoned to carrying the moral stigma of 'child killer'. Moreover, if in doubt about which is the correct decision, they will turn to doctors for more than advice — for absolution, for guidance and possibly even for direction. Yet they will carry the personal burden of having apparently made the decision in the exercise of this elusive "choice".

The modern face of medical science poses, therefore, a further threat to women's exercise of autonomy. By leaping into the dark, by asking questions where the answers (and indeed the questions themselves) are laden with hidden agendas and assumptions, yet again the medical profession becomes the central predictor of abortion decisions. So, what role is there for the law here?

If, as has been suggested in the theme of this book, we look to the law to guide and control influences which may limit or remove human rights, and if — as Petersen suggests[38] — no legal model yet devised has actually achieved this in the case of abortion, does not the whole edifice on which this book is premised collapse?

The answer must be 'no'. A presumption that the law can and should regulate the access of citizens to human rights does not inevitably require direct legal intervention. In fact, on the premise that 'less is more', there may well be occasions when direct legal comment is inappropriate. It is an accepted part of legal analysis that what is not prohibited is prima facie permitted. In this situation, **removing** laws which govern abortion may well be the most proactive strike which law can make. To be sure, it would not prevent the influences which already exist in society from informing the ultimate decision as to whether or not to continue with a pregnancy, but it would deny them the overt backing of the law. In addition, law can play a tangential but important function by helping to shape a society which assists those faced with difficult decisions to make the one which is best suited to them rather than the one which seems the most obvious. Women may seek genetic and other information about the health of their foetus but, as Dworkin has pointed out, a society which really values their choice would make it genuinely free by removing from it the anxieties which follow from it.[39]

Women take pregnancy and parenting seriously — in fact, it is precisely because of this that abortion decisions should be available. The decision to end a pregnancy is one which is also taken seriously, and which should be available with the minimum of external pressure. Truly liberal laws would not intrude into this private choice, not even on the pretext of the state's interest in the embryo or foetus. This is not to say that the product of conception can be simply dismissed as completely irrelevant, but it is a challenge to current thinking. There is no inherent paradox in respecting the embryo or foetus while at the same time accepting that the choice of a competent person to terminate a pregnancy is worthy of the kind of respect which it is currently denied. By demanding medical involvement, or by claiming that third parties (for example, the state) have an interest in the foetus which can override that of the person carrying it, women and their decisions are infantilised and devalued.

The paradox of this situation is mirrored in the other main consequence of medicalising pregnancy — namely the additional pressure which may now be brought on women — not to continue with a pregnancy but to terminate it in the interests of 'inter-generational justice'. The choice in favour of, rather than against, the continuation of a pregnancy is becoming equally medicalised and sometimes categorised as selfish, particularly where it is known that the child will not be born 'normal'. Moreover, the real ability to decide to continue with such a pregnancy may be inhibited, if not precluded, by the failure of the state (through the law) to provide the facilities which help women to cope with the consequences of their choice. If women are to be free to make a real choice, a range of options must be available. The reality at the moment is that the choice to end or to continue with a preg-nancy is constrained. Women are in a position where they cannot win.

It is central to this argument that women must be permitted to make decisions to terminate or continue with a pregnancy, subject to the scrutiny only of their own consciences and not — however subtly — controlled by the morals of doctors. This inevitably means that decisions will be made for a wide variety of reasons — from the totally selfish to the altruistic. But free-dom in this, as in other areas, demands that the exercise of autonomy is not predicated on others understanding or endors-ing our decision. Yet, in this most personal of matters, the unthinking absorption of medical influence and scientific cant has reduced a matter of human rights to one of medical monopoly. The collusion of the law is, as in so many other cases, to be deeply regretted.

5 Controlling Fertility
The Case of Mentally Disabled People

Reproduction has come to occupy a central position in the theatre of the personal. It has moved upstage, from being seen as a minor bit part of personhood, to being cast as one of the essential characteristics of its successful production and realisation.[1]

As earlier chapters have shown, reproductive liberty is one of the major values which we claim to take seriously. But throughout the centuries, reproductive liberties — particularly those claimed by women — have been at the centre of fierce political, social and legal debate. From the early attempts to limit the availability of freely obtainable contraception and abortion, through early twentieth-century eugenics programmes, to modern, assisted reproductive technologies, reproductive choice has been both controlled and controversial. Society seems to be somewhat ambivalent about just what freedoms women should have in deciding whether or not to have children.

There is one group for whom our approach to reproductive liberty is peculiarly important; namely mentally disabled people. The uncertainty about what rights women in general have concerning their own fertility is compounded when the individual concerned is believed to lack the legal capacity to decide for herself. The existence of disability can be used in two critical ways.

First, it may be used to disvalue the intuitions and feelings of the disabled person, and second — in a more extreme way — it may provide an apparent rationale for the use of compulsion. This second issue will be considered in more depth later.

There is an apparently widespread perception that the fact of mental disability logically means that those afflicted will not experience pregnancy and childbirth in the same way as others, and that they will inevitably be unable to care for a child. As Shaw, for example, has said, 'The supposed absence of maternal feelings in mentally disabled women, their assumed inability to care for any offspring and the pain that they might suffer if they were separated from a child are common themes in recent English cases although in the absence of definable criteria for decision-making it is hard to tell what weight is placed upon them.'[2] As will be seen later, these presumptions have also informed the jurisprudence of other countries.

But where is the evidence that they are actually true? Reliance on the clinical assessment of capacity has led courts in many countries to agree to non-consensual sterilisations for reasons which are, in some cases, highly dubious. It is perhaps trite to note that we do not subject 'normal' women to such tests (although for many of them pregnancy, childbirth and parenting are difficult), but it is not fatuous to question the grounds on which such assumptions are made about, and used against, disabled people. Even more worrying is the ready acceptance by courts that evidence of handicap provides a basis for a wide-ranging set of conclusions which need not follow from that diagnosis — most particularly that childbearing should be avoided. The consequence of this presumption has been the use of sterilisation as an effective way of avoiding pregnancy and childbirth. Too often, this is based on the assumption that somehow disabled people, because of their disability, will not feel deprived of the capacity to become pregnant or the opportunity to parent in the same way as 'normal' women would. This belief seems to be widespread, although it is based on no real empirical evidence.

The Law Reform Commission of Canada, for example, undertook extensive research into this issue and concluded, 'It has been found that, like anyone else, the mentally handicapped have individually varying reactions to sterilisation. Sex and parenthood hold the same significance for them as for other people .... The psychological impact of sterilisation is likely to be particularly damaging in cases where it is the result of coercion and when mentally disabled people have had no children.'[3]

In a Canadian judgement,[4] which has largely been dismissed in UK cases, La Forest pointed to a very significant factor in decisions of this sort. Rather than seeing the decision as being critically informed by clinical judgement or the welfare of others, his view was that the basis for decision-making should reflect other values and be cautious about over-intrusion. As he said, 'The argument relating to fitness to parent involves many value-loaded questions ... there are human rights considerations that should make a court extremely hesitant about attempting to solve a social problem like this by this means.'[5]

Deprivation of the capacity to have children is undoubtedly a human rights issue, and one which must be taken seriously. As long ago as 1971 the United Nations declared that — in as much as it was possible — the disabled should be accorded the same rights as other citizens. International[6] and European[7] Declarations endorsed the centrality of the family, and the right to marry and found a family within existing national laws. As La Forest has said, 'The importance of maintaining the physical integrity of a human being ranks high in our scale of values, particularly as it affects the privilege of giving life.'[8] Without clear and convincing evidence to the contrary, therefore, one might reasonably assume that decisions authorising non-consensual sterilisation would be taken only rarely and with utmost concern for the rights of those affected. Such an expectation, would, however, be too simplistic.

To an extent, it is difficult not to conclude that our recent history continues to inform our present decision-making. La Forest has said, 'There are other reasons for approaching an application for sterilisation of a mentally incompetent person with the utmost caution. To begin with, the decision involves values in an area where our social history clouds our vision and encourages many to perceive the mentally handicapped as somewhat less than human.'[9] Although it is now likely that cases will come before courts — at least where there is a dispute about whether or not sterilisation should proceed — there may none the less be subliminal assumptions incorporated into the matter and evidence presented which render the court process less than effective.

The terms of the UN Declaration demand due process for mentally disabled people, but this is not satisfied merely by a court hearing the case. In such serious and complex matters, justice is only served where the criteria used in the decision-making process are themselves stringent and set clearly and unequivocally against a backdrop of respect for rights. The preliminary presumption must, therefore, be that rights should not be removed unless there is a real and demonstrable need for this. Despite the conflicting evidence available, it is not always clear that consideration of anything other than the medical recommendation is undertaken, and it is certainly true that reported cases do not accurately reflect the number of sterilisations which are being undertaken at the instigation of those who care for mentally disabled people. In a recent Scottish case,[10] for example, the judge noted that there had been previous cases involving non-consensual sterilisation in which authority had been granted to proceed without any formal

opposition. This case was the first in which there was opposition
to the granting of the authority. Without knowing how many cases
had been permitted before, it is scarcely reassuring that the first
case in which the decision was challenged in this jurisdiction was
heard in 1996.

What can be concluded, then, is that decisions are being taken
in a number of cases with adversion only to the medical evidence
and with reference to the wishes of the carers. That these may be
fallible is ably demonstrated by the English case of *Re D*[11] and the
Canadian case of *Re Eve*.[12] In *Re D*, the sterilisation of an 11-year-
old had been agreed by her mother and her doctor. A concerned
third party succeeded in getting the case heard in court, and
authority for the sterilisation was denied. The young woman in
question was thought likely to improve and likely to be legally
able to marry when of an age to do so. Heilbron described the
proposed surgery as 'the deprivation of a basic human right,
namely the right of a woman to reproduce...'.[13] Interestingly, the
judge was prepared to fly in the face of the medical recommendation saying, 'I cannot believe, and the evidence does not warrant
the view, that a decision to carry out an operation of this nature
performed for non-therapeutic purposes on a minor, can be held
to be within the doctor's sole clinical judgment.'[14]

In *Re Eve,* the court also drew attention to the human rights
issues involved, and paid special attention to the purpose of the
sterilisation. It was, as La Forest said, 'admittedly non-therapeutic'.[15] That is, it was designed to avoid pregnancy and not to
alleviate a clinical condition. The woman concerned was an adult,
whose elderly mother feared that she might become pregnant and
felt unable to care for any child which her daughter might have.
Despite the sympathy which the court showed to the mother, the
judge concluded that, 'The grave intrusion on a person's rights
and the certain physical damage that ensues from non-therapeu-

tic sterilisation without consent, when compared to the highly questionable advantages that can result from it, have persuaded me that it can never safely be determined that such a procedure is for the benefit of the person'.[16]

If the reasoning in these cases formed the basis for decision-making then it might be felt that the rights of disabled people would be afforded adequate protection. Unfortunately this has not routinely proved to be the case. The congruence of medical recommendation with socially constructed bias has, on the contrary, often downgraded the reproductive liberties of mentally disabled people and restricted their freedoms, with no clear rationale or consistent application of principles. As Shaw points out,

> Strikingly different solutions to similar problems are often adopted: there is, for instance, no consensus among judges, legislators and other policy makers on recourse to or rejection of non-consensual sterilisation as an appropriate technological response to the social 'problem' of sexual activity by those unable by reason of mental disability to conform to the norms and demands of modern society ...[17]

To an extent, this lack of cohesive and clear policies is a result of the reluctance of decision-makers to challenge medical recommendations and the trepidation with which mentally disabled people are approached. This century has seen widespread abuse of the disabled (amongst others) in the name of medical 'knowledge'. In countries as disparate as the United States and Nazi Germany, medicine and politics combined to provide a powerful machinery which overwhelmed the rights of certain groups, disabled people among them.[18]

The impetus for this came from the emerging science of genetics. Relying on Mendelian principles, scientists came to see that certain characteristics were inherited through the genes. In itself, this might be taken to be unobjectionable, although there are reasons to be concerned about even the 'new' genetics which I will discuss later. In the wrong hands, however, scientific knowledge became a vehicle for compulsion. Working on the assumption that all characteristics were inherited, and sure in the knowledge of which characteristics were unwanted, the United States embarked upon a policy of compulsory sterilisation of the 'undesirable'.

By the 1930s, a number of American States had enacted legislation permitting the involuntary sterilisation of certain groups, and in a number of cases these statutes stayed on the statute books for many years afterwards. In Germany, hundreds of thousands of 'undesirables' were sterilised in the vanguard of the politics of hatred. But underlying all of this was the force of science. Seen as a value-free and accurate discipline, it provided the perfect rationale for the deprivation of rights. Equally, scientists and doctors were active in turning their elementary genetic knowledge into political platforms and legal controls. The force of science has seldom been more clearly demonstrated, and its most powerful exposition comes from the United States case of *Buck* v. *Bell*[19] and the judgement of Oliver Wendell Holmes briefly referred to earlier. Convinced by medical evidence that the young woman concerned was 'feeble minded', and that her mother and daughter were 'feeble-minded' also, he authorised non-consensual sterilisation and held it not to be unconstitutional. His rationale was as follows:

> We have seen more than once that the public welfare may call upon the best citizens for their lives. It would be strange if it could not call upon those who already sap the strength of the State for these lesser sacrifices, often not felt to be

such by those concerned, in order to prevent our being swamped with incompetence. It is better for all the world, if instead of waiting to execute degenerate offspring for crime, or to let them starve for their imbecility, society can prevent those who are manifestly unfit from continuing their kind. The principle that sustains compulsory vaccination is broad enough to cover cutting the Fallopian tubes .... Three generations of imbeciles are enough.[20]

This quotation shows most starkly how science can knowingly as well as unknowingly be used as a tool of oppression. It was not until the case of *Skinner* v. *Oklahoma*[21] in 1942 that Douglas said 'marriage and procreation are fundamental to the very existence and survival of the race. The power to sterilise, if exercised, may have subtle, far-reaching and devastating effects. In evil or reckless hands it can cause races or types which are inimical to the dominant group to wither and disappear.'[22]

The history of abuse during the early part of this century is well documented and does not require further elaboration here. But the lessons to be learned from it are more than historical. Norrie has said that, 'The mentally disabled are as entitled to enjoy sexual relations as the rest of us, subject only to their requiring protection from exploitation.'[23] Leaving aside the question of whether or not disabled people are the only group vulnerable to exploitation, he makes a telling point. The rights which we are talking about here are bigger than any alleged 'right' to reproduce. They are not simply about people's reproductive organs but rather about the physical inviolability of the individual. Certainly, those fortunate enough not to be disabled might well conclude that we are best served when our rights to bodily integrity are respected, including our capacity to procreate. There is no reason to presume that these desires should not equally inform our approach to disabled people.

If, therefore, it can be concluded that mentally disabled people should be free to act upon their sexuality in the same way as anyone else, then it might be expected that the state would have no role to play in controlling this. Certainly, as Norrie says, we may wish to protect people from exploitation, but it is equally clear that sterilising them does not achieve this. In fact, removing the risk of pregnancy might make disabled people even more vulnerable to sexual exploitation. This is not to say that protection is out of place. An element of paternalism in respect of the vulnerable is a common characteristic of developed legal systems. We routinely seek to protect children and other groups, and there is no reason why we should not also try to protect those whose capacity for judgement may be in other ways reduced. As Dickens says, 'not all paternalism is offensive or an insult to autonomy'.[24]

However, some forms of paternalism undoubtedly are, and the reasons given for exercising paternalism are not always convincing. Legitimate paternalism would undoubtedly include protection from abuse, but, in the case of disabled people, this is attainable only by the provision of the kind of community in which they are free to exercise their rights to the fullest without fear of predators. Sterilisation does not mean that they will not be vulnerable to sexual assault, unsuitable liaisons or sexually transmitted diseases. All that it does is to ensure that no conception takes place, reinforcing the earlier suggestion that the actual reasons for non-consensual sterilisations are not the same as those which are overtly given.

Undoubtedly, attitudes have changed. There is an increasing desire to facilitate the integration of disabled people into the community, but as has been suggested this desire is by no means absolute. Commenting on the UK case of *F* v. *Berkshire Health Authority*,[25] Shaw makes the following telling point:

The sexuality of mentally disabled persons, like any other aspect of sexual behaviour, is a socially constructed phenomenon. That mentally disabled people are increasingly accorded the physical and emotional space within which to realise their sexual urges and needs is not the consequence of a new biological imperative but of a shift in the boundaries of what is regarded as socially acceptable conduct. Yet we have only come so far in the lifting of taboos and the redefinition of social acceptability. We may be at ease with the sexual activity of F and others like her, but we make her freedom a conditional freedom: conception must be avoided at all costs.[26]

This, then, is not in fact about the avoidance of exploitation. Rather, it is an incorporation into medical and legal thinking of presumptions about the capacity of some women to cope with pregnancy, childbirth and parenting — presumptions which have already been shown to be at best ill founded and at worst demeaning. Moreover, these assumptions also disguise different, but equally discriminatory, prejudices. In Canada, for example, it has been noted that, 'in dealing with such serious issues, provincial sterilisation boards have revealed serious differences in their attitudes as between men and women, the poor and the rich, and people of different ethnic backgrounds...'.[27] That these same characteristics are also visible in cases of forced obstetrical intervention suggests that they, rather than the condition or interests of the woman, are critical to decisions which result in the minimisation of rights.

Before considering contemporary attitudes to the sterilisation of mentally disabled people, it is, however, worth making one further point. It cannot be argued, and I do not intend to argue, that sterilisation of mentally disabled people is never permissible or that it is always a denial of rights. If I have the right to sterilisation, as I do, then so too should the mentally disabled, a point made clear in the US case of *Re Grady*.[28] We must be careful not the deny people something which others can freely attain. But the test of a civilised society is that it does protect the vulnerable from unnecessary and unwarranted invasion. To move too far in either direction would be equally obnoxious, but we must err, if erring there is, on the side of challenging our own presuppositions and in favour of the approach based on respect for persons. Lee and Morgan argue that:

> Against such recent histories of the use of sterilisation for overtly eugenic purposes, the stance of courts at least in the United States as bulwarks against the proposed sterilisations is so dominant that it is seriously argued that the difficulties in obtaining sterilisation for the mentally disabled infringes their freedom to choose an appropriate contraceptive regime.[29]

However, they conclude that 'In Britain an entirely contrary danger is apparent'.[30]

Even if Lee and Morgan are right in their assessment of the dangers of the US situation, in other countries the real threat is posed by the too ready assumption that the existence of handicap is *in se* enough to justify differential treatment. In these countries the capacity of disabled people to live a full life is constrained by the too easy enthusiasm for non-consensual sterilisation on the basis of presumption not fact. In the UK, for example, despite the cautious and thoughtful decisions in *Re D* and *Re Eve*, there is little doubt that judges have followed the same path as they generally do — namely, that they will by and large endorse the recommendations of the clinicians and the families of people with disablility. Indeed, a review of some of the recent cases suggests that courts have been much more exercised about whether or not they have the power to make sterilisation decisions than they have been about the reasons for making them.

Of course, this is not to deny that there has been considerable debate about the basis on which such decisions can be made — that is, what are the legal tests to be applied when such a serious decision is contemplated. Identification of the appropriate test could, of course, go some long way towards the protection of rights and it is therefore important that considerable energy should be expended on describing, defining and delimiting it.

Broadly speaking, courts have available to them two main tests: the substituted judgement test and the best interests test. The first attempts:

> to determine what decision the mental incompetent would make, if she was reviewing her situation as a competent person, but taking account of her mental incapacity as one factor in her decision. It allows the court to consider a number of factors bearing directly on the condition of the mental incompetent .... In essence, an attempt is made to determine the actual interests and preferences of the mental incompetent. This, it is thought, recognises her moral dignity and right to free choice. [31]

However, as a tool for use in this kind of situation, substituted judgement has obvious flaws.

Since the person has usually never been competent, at best this test becomes intelligent guesswork, subject to the same subliminal incorporation of bias as any other test would be. Although a useful test in situations where it is possible to identify what values a person may previously have prioritised, it is probably unsuited to cases where competence has never been present. However, it does have some value in that it seems to place direct attention on the individual herself. But it is subject to the fundamental flaw that evidence about the individual's wishes must still come from third parties, for example parents or doctors, whose interests — however caring — may realistically be expected, at least on some occasions, to be divergent from those of the woman herself.

However, some jurisdictions have found the test to be useful. As Mason notes, in the United States, 'Effectively, *Grady* introduced a "substituted judgment" test which allows for full consideration of the incompetent's right to choose through the medium of his or her parents.'[32] In laying down strict criteria, as did the slightly earlier case of *Re Hayes*,[33] the court in *Grady*[34] undoubtedly made non-consensual sterilisation more difficult, but they also recognised that it was necessary actually to test both the fact of incompetence and the relative weight to be given to the risks of pregnancy and childbirth as against the damage which could be caused by sterilisation. The sensitivity of US courts to the underlying human rights issues may well be a direct result of their recent history, and some courts have shown themselves to be reluctant to make the decision asked. As was said in *Re Guardianship of Tully*,[35] 'the awesome power to deprive a human being of his or her fundamental right to bear or beget offspring must be founded on the explicit authorisation by the Legislature...'[36] In *Re Guardianship of Eberhardy*,[37] J. Hefferman, said:

> courts, even by taking judicial notice of medical treatises, know very little of the techniques or efficacy of contraceptive methods or of thwarting the ability to procreate by methods short of sterilisation. While courts are always dependent upon the opinions of expert witnesses, it would appear that the exercise of judicial discretion unguided by well-thought-out policy determinations reflecting the

interests of society, as well as of the person to be sterilised, are hazardous indeed.[38]

In other words, these are very difficult decisions and whether or not they are made by judges or legislatures they require careful analysis of a wide range of complex interests and issues. Nonetheless, it seems to be common ground that sometimes these decisions will have to be taken, although not always by a court. However, those cases which do reach a court provide us with the clearest available signals about the extent to which the rights and interests of the disabled are actually being respected. Given the acknowledged shortcomings of the substituted judgement test, the majority approach has been to adopt a 'best interests' test.

Now, of course, this test — essentially a welfare test — is the one commonly used in dealing with persons who are not deemed legally capable of reaching their own decisions. It is one, therefore, with which the courts are relatively familiar and comfortable, but for all that Norrie suggests it 'suffers from being amorphous and unpredictable. Of its nature, it has to be subjective, but this allows for different courts to take different views as to what course of action will be best.'[39] Not only this, but it permits yet again of inbuilt prejudice dominating the decision. Although opting for a best interests test in *Re Eve*,[40] La Forest sought to refine it by distinguishing between therapeutic and non-therapeutic sterilisation. The former could be accommodated under the welfare principle while the latter could not. Referring to the earlier Canadian case of *Re K and Public Trustee*[41] he also drew attention to the need for careful definition of what was in fact therapeutic. In this case, the Court of Appeal of British Columbia ordered a hysterectomy to be carried out on a retarded child who was said to have a phobic reaction to blood, and for whom menstruation was thought to be ill-advised. Although the judge in that case said, 'I say now, as forcefully as I can, this case cannot and must not be regarded as a precedent to be followed in cases involving sterilisation of mentally disabled persons for contraceptive purposes',[42] La Forest described the judgement as being 'at best dangerously close to the limits of the permissible'.[43]

It might be thought that some of the problems of the best interests test could be alleviated by the adoption of La Forest's distinction between therapeutic and non-therapeutic, even granted that the line may sometimes be difficult to draw clearly. Certainly, adopting this distinction would seem to rule out non-consensual sterilisations which are for social rather than health-related reasons and would put a welcome brake on medical and legal discretion. However, this has not commended itself to British courts, despite Lord Brandon's definition of best interests as being treatment 'carried out either to save their lives, or to ensure improvement or prevent deterioration in their physical or mental health'.[44] This statement would seem to suggest that medical health was the critical indicator for sterilisation, corresponding fairly closely to the distinction made by La Forest, although as Ogbourne and Ward point out, 'It is difficult to conceive of medical treatment (other, perhaps, than some treatments of a cosmetic nature) which do not literally fall within this formulation'.[45]

In the case of *Re B*,[46] however, Lord Bridge dismissed La Forest's reasoning.

> This sweeping generalisation seems to me, with respect, to be entirely unhelpful. To say that the court can never authorise sterilisation of a ward as being in her best interests would be patently wrong. To say that it can only do so if the operation is 'therapeutic' as opposed to 'non-therapeutic' is to divert attention from the true issue, which is whether the

operation is in the ward's best interest, and remove it to an area of arid semantic debate as to where the line is to be drawn'.[47]

Strong words indeed but the question remains, have he and his colleagues come up with a better or more satisfactory definition? Sadly, the answer must be no. UK courts have shown themselves to be concerned to identify the relevant test — best interests — without fleshing it out. In many of the cases, it is in fact clear that the 'best interests' test will be met where there is a congruence of clinical recommendation, parental support and judicial inclination. The reported cases have shown, as has been seen, that the medical willingness to sterilise, especially when coupled with parental approval, has been a critical predictor of the outcome, even if the woman is not in a sexual relationship and her fertility has never been assessed.

A number of UK cases give cause for concern. In the case of *Re B*,[48] for example, although Lord Dillon indicated that the power to authorise sterilisation should 'be exercised only in the last resort',[49] his colleague, Lord Oliver, clearly saw the human rights issues in a different way. Indeed, his assertion that 'the right to reproduce is of value only if accompanied by the ability to make a choice',[50] is eerily and unhappily reminiscent of the judgement in *Buck v. Bell*. In any event, if awareness or ability to make a choice were central to the exercise of a right or to its preservation, then many rights, such as the right to life, would be defeated by mental handicap or the fact of unconsciousness. This, I am sure, no judge would argue, and the suspicion lurks that the use of the argument in non-consensual sterilisation cases is merely a mask for the fact that the judge did not feel that it was appropriate for this person to reproduce, or that reproductive freedoms and capacities were somehow less important for that person.

Perhaps inevitably, the UK courts have also depended heavily, as is their wont, on the *Bolam* test.[51] This test uses acceptable medical practice as a yardstick of whether or not the operation in question was properly carried out. But the test is designed to judge the **competence** of a medical procedure — it is not designed to test its **lawfulness,** and it is therefore entirely inappropriate in such cases. As Ogbourne and Ward say, 'The fact that the majority of medical judgement may arrive at a particular decision tells us no more than that the practitioner is following accepted practice. It does not tell us whether that practice is right. That is surely a function of the courts.'[52] And as Brazier points out, 'For the woman, if the Bolam test and the Bolam test alone establishes the lawfulness of surgery then judicial intervention does little more than protect her from the complete maverick whom none of his colleagues would back in his decision to sterilise her.'[53]

Two other cases, *Re M*[54] and *Re P*[55] introduced one further consideration — that of reversibility. Both are of concern, but perhaps *Re P* is the more worrying of the two. In this case, the woman in question was said to have a mental age of six, but her communication skills were good and improving. The court recognised that she might have some maternal feelings, but her mother was afraid that if she did become pregnant she would not agree to an abortion. It was said that, for the moment, she regarded intercourse as painful and that she was not therefore at risk of pregnancy and that she might well value the 'right' to reproduce. At least some of the characteristics which are often said to be absent in people with mental disability, therefore, were admittedly present in this case. Nonetheless, the judge authorised the sterilisation and was clearly heavily influenced by the evidence of an eminent specialist that the operation had a 95 per cent chance of being reversible.

Just what this tells us about judicial attitudes to removal of reproductive choice is instructive. Even although there was no current assessed risk of pregnancy and even although this 17 year old might well have valued childbearing in precisely the same way as any other young woman, major surgery was used as a form of contraception, presumably on the grounds that in reality the court didn't think she was the 'right' kind of person to breed. The notion of reversibility is a convenient disguise for what seems on the face of it to be a decision based on prejudice against people with mental disability informed by little if any evidence and in flagrant disregard of the importance to women of reproductive capacity. As Brazier says, 'He [the judge] is in effect saying to P that because there is available the technology to reverse her sterilisation, the initial decision to sterilise may be taken more lightly, albeit the actual chances of her obtaining a reversal operation are minimal and that the operation, if undertaken, would be attended by greater risk and discomfort to her than the original surgery.'[56]

Of further concern in this case, as in some of the others, is the tacit concession that the woman in question might not in fact **be** incapable of making her own decision in the future. But the authority of the court to substitute its judgement for that of the woman only arises if it is clear that she is and will continue to be incompetent. Brazier concludes, 'The judgements in *Re M* and *Re P* do not inspire confidence in the judiciary's readiness to develop and apply clear guidelines defining competence.'[57]

One further point needs to be mentioned. Throughout these cases one very obvious question is conspicuous by its absence — namely, are the women concerned fertile? Whether or not they are engaged in, or are likely to be engaged in, sexual relationships is the subject of much speculation, but their actual capacity to reproduce is not tested. Given that there is some evidence that people with severe disability are less fertile than others in the community, might this not be a relevant consideration? Lord MacLean in a recent Scottish case noted that he had not been invited to consider this matter and remarked, 'It is remarkable how frequently in litigation central issues or critical considerations are overlooked or not identified.'[58] Remarkable indeed, but scarcely reassuring.

This brief review of some of the important cases reveals some worrying phenomena. Arguably, we have not yet reached the point where we are prepared to regard people with mental disability as full citizens, possessed of rights and worthy of respect. Moreover, the cavalier attitude of many judges to the inherently significant interest of the individual in reproductive liberty reflects a cultural bias which is, once exposed, distasteful. Despite repeated assertions that these decisions are not based on eugenic grounds, that they are designed to prevent exploitation and that they are for the benefit of the women themselves, analysis suggests that they may, rather, reflect a deeper and more sinister reality.

And Freeman[59] is concerned that there is an inexorable logic to these decisions which might start us down a slippery slope. As he says, 'Once rights are "trumped" on the ground that it is for the right-holder's own good, it is but a simple step to argue that a right should also be undermined where to do so is for the good of others or the general good.'[60] His concern is that the pattern may come full circle and return us to the days when people with disability (and others) were seen as pawns in a larger social plan, with few rights and limited protections. Whether or not this is a logical outcome, it is a salient concern worth bearing in mind.

There is good reason to be anxious about the way in which some courts have approached the non-consensual removal of reproductive liberties from women with disability. Analysis of the judgements shows legal incoherence in the face of medical 'fact'. It is one thing to accept a medical assessment of intelligence or a psychological profile of skills or to agree in certain peculiarly difficult situations that sterilisation is necessary in the best inter-

ests of the woman. It is quite another to conclude that best interests are definable by medical or parental or even judicial
preferences. We may have moved from overt eugenics, but we do
not yet seem to have made the final leap towards valuing for others
what we value for ourselves.

As Gillon says:

> Our attitudes to proposals for the sterilisation of mentally
> handicapped people are subject to powerful emotions —
> emotions that influence our responses to sexuality in general,
> emotions that influence our responses to mental handicap
> in general, and emotions that are heightened by our attitudes
> to a society whose morality functions as a dread warning of
> the depths to which human behaviour can sink. In such
> circumstances we must be even more than usually meticu-
> lous about subjecting our 'gut response' to the searchlight
> of critical moral reasoning.[61]

These are wise words, but in reality this 'searchlight' also requires
enlightenment. Not just enlightenment of our attitude to the
disabled, but enlightenment as to the fundamental issues involved
in such decisions. It is not enough that non-consensual sterilisations receive the endorsement of a court. The payment of lip-service
to due process of the law does not ensure that the decisions made
are reached for good reasons and with due regard to human
rights. Concentration on the use of reproductive organs alone
disvalues the person. It may be that some, even all, of the women
who have been sterilised would indeed have suffered as a result
of pregnancy and/or childbirth but, as Brazier puts it, 'Pregnancy
is a disaster for all too many women. Yet no one suggests that all
women likely to be incapable of coping with childbirth and/or
child care should be forcibly sterilised.'[62]

Nor can we hide behind the claim that we are simply protecting the vulnerable. By sterilising these women we do not reduce — may even increase — their risk of sexual exploitation. We do violence to them and to their rights without having adequately considered what might be their **real** interests. There is, and must be, a role for the law to play, but it must rise above dependence on outmoded assumptions and medical 'certainties'. Moreover, it must and should address its aspirations to protect the individual against the invasive behaviour of others. The half-hearted attempts to justify non-consensual sterilisations do not stand up to rigorous scrutiny in more than a few cases. We must be cautious not to deprive people with disability of the right not to become pregnant, but just as importantly we must be satisfied that sterilisation **is** only used as a last resort and does not become a means of appeasing others whose interests are not the same as those of the women concerned, no matter how well intentioned. Only a legal system independent of over-reliance on clinical judgement and sensitive to human rights is capable of achieving this.

This section of the book has concentrated on reproductive issues. The emphasis on reproduction is inevitable because it is here that much of what it is to be human rests and here that liberties are particularly at risk. However, the collusion of law and medicine is equally apparent at the end of life also, and it is to this area that I will now turn.

6 The Infant with Disability
To Treat or Not to Treat?

Medicine can influence they way we live in a variety of ways. Some of them may be purposive and clear, but others are more subtle. Much of what follows in the next chapters is concerned with the latter but the fundamental concerns remain similar. Medical advances often result in new and sometimes tragic dilemmas being raised — dilemmas which we may be ill-equipped to address. The problems posed are often complex and none more so than when considering what should or should not be done in respect of infants born with severe handicaps.

This is not a new problem, but it is one which has changed shape over the years. As Smith points out, 'Although generally considered unlawful, non-treatment of disabled newborns is probably not a rare event. One study, for example, found that 14 per cent of all infant deaths in the studied hospital were related to withdrawal or withholding of medical treatment.'[1] In the past, decisions about whether or not to offer treatment were taken in private, leading Wells to say that the issue is 'not only dimly lit but is hardly on the stage at all'.[2] More recently, however, some high-profile cases have brought the question of selective non-treatment on to centre stage as one of our most difficult contemporary ethical dilemmas. This is so despite the impact of medicine as well as because of it. On the one hand, many disabilities can be identified pre-birth allowing parents the opportunity of deciding whether or not to continue with the pregnancy. On the other hand, not every condition can be tested for, not every woman is prepared to have tests undertaken and advances in neonatal therapy mean that

> low birth weight and disabled children may now be saved, whereas some years ago they would certainly have died. The dilemma, then, is what should medicine do and who should have the authority to make the decision.

It has been estimated by Shapiro that, 'Each year, approximately 30,000 severely defective babies are born in the United States.'[3] This is a small but significant percentage of live births, and occurs despite sophisticated screening programmes. But far from presuming that, once born, these babies are entitled to all the treatment which is available, choices have been, and are, made about which should be treated and which not. These decisions may be based on a number of factors — personal, ethical or economic. And they are made despite the fact that treatment may be available which would maintain existence. As Whitelaw says

> Neonatal intensive-care units have the ability to prolong the lives of infants with profound neurological abnormalities, including some who will never enjoy independent meaningful lives. Furthermore, neonatal intensive care is an expensive and scarce resource which is sometimes denied to viable infants because of shortages of nurses or equipment. Against this background, many paediatricians have practised selection in applying high-technology life-support techniques.[4]

Unsurprisingly, feelings run high about these practices, now that they are in the public domain. The issues to be resolved are not merely technical, nor in theory should they be dependent on the availability of resources. Unless we are to treat these infants as non-people, it is essential that a coherent framework for decision making is identified. This also demands that the decision maker is unbiased and accountable. In the past, however, severe cases were dealt with primarily by doctors and generally in private. As Campbell and Duff say, 'Traditionally, doctors alone made a decision for or against treatment, often without any reference to parental views in the well-meaning but mistaken belief that they were sparing grief-stricken parents an unbearable additional burden'.[5]

Whether or not doctors should make such decisions will be dealt with in more depth later, but for the moment it is worth noting that there are strongly held differences of opinion on whether or not such decisions should be made at all. For Robertson, 'The pervasive practice of withholding ordinary medical care from defective newborns demonstrates that we have embarked on a widespread practice of involuntary euthanasia'.[6] For others, failing to salvage lives whose quality will be poor is both justifiable and compassionate. Clearly, the answer to the question as to whether or not such decisions should be made will depend on the ethical standpoint of those who seek to answer it. Since it logically precedes the question of who should make the decision, it must be considered first.

As Mason has said, 'The possibility that heroic treatment of the defective neonate may be ill-conceived has been apparent for many years and essentially focuses on the problem of whether the doctor's function is to preserve life at all costs or to improve the quality of life.'[7] For some, the answer is clear. All human life is sacred and every effort should be made to preserve it. Of course, some infants will be born terminally ill and the question here is different. Where no therapy can help, the law has generally conceded that only comfort care is necessary. But the group who are of most concern are those infants who may live (for a short or a long time) in pain or discomfort or who will survive never to interact with those around them.

As societies we claim to take the sanctity of life very seriously. It has been said that 'No viable society can afford to allow for any but the most *absolutely necessary exceptions* to the prohibition against one individual taking the life of another.'[8] By implication, if that line were followed, no one should allow a child in their care to die either. In other words, life should be protected as a rule whose violation demands strictly controlled and narrowly drawn exceptions. As one commentator says, 'Basing life and death decisions on physical or mental abnormalities is inconsistent with the belief that human life should be protected without regard to status or defects.'[9]

Despite the problems with a sanctity of life argument (not least that we tend to be somewhat inconsistent in our application of it and that we circumscribe it with escape clauses) McLean and Maher described it as 'emotionally appealing' and the 'simplest' approach to these dilemmas.[10] 'The belief that life is sacred logically implies that all life, even if damaged, merits equal and total protection. One of the immediate charms of this argument is that it is overtly non-discriminatory ...'[11]

Discrimination is undoubtedly a real fear. Decisions based on quality of life rather than on the existence of life itself, undoubtedly permit the incorporation of individual and collective bias. Although it has been said that 'There is no principle of law which distinguishes the care due to a mentally defective infant from that due to one who is normal',[12] it is clear that differences are drawn. For the child who is born needing therapy but likely to live a relatively 'normal' life, the only constraint on providing the treatment would be resource based. By and large these children will be treated and their lives saved. However, unarguably, the graver the defect the less likely it is that the child will be treated.

Nor is it necessary that the clinical condition of the child is particularly severe before such decisions may be made. For example,
'one study revealed that 85 per cent of the paediatric surgeons
and 65 per cent of the paediatricians surveyed would be willing
to honour parental wishes not to perform necessary surgery on
a Down's syndrome child, but less than 6 per cent would deny
similar treatment for a child without the disability'.[13] What is being
taken into account here is a combination of parental attitudes, clinicians' views and the anticipated quality of life of the child. The
first two of these will be dealt with later, but the notion of quality of life being used as a life or death predictor concerns many
people.

Some would argue that quality of life decisions should never
be made, that they are morally wrong and technically uncertain.
As Rhoden points out, 'Withholding treatment based on quality
of life decisions has been roundly condemned by many courts and
legal commentators and has been deemed nearly as reprehensi-
ble as denying care to an infant born in a ghetto because it is likely
to grow up in poverty, ignorance and squalor.'[14] And it is equally
true that some babies, whose initial clinical prognosis was poor,
have gone on to astound the experts and to live fulfilled and
fulfilling lives. Even as medicine becomes more accurate in terms
of prognosis there will still be cases in which it will be proved
wrong, a further argument likely to commend itself to those for
whom the sanctity of life is paramount.

Even those who are not fully committed to the view that all
human life is sacred may be concerned about quality of life decisions, based, as they often are, on ignorance of the condition itself
and its impact on the individual. Glanville Williams's[15] comments
following two English cases doubtless shocked many, as well as
pointing to the difficulties of making decisions of this sort on behalf
of others. He said, 'If a wicked fairy told me that she was about

to transform me into a Down's baby (or a Down's adult) and asked me whether in these circumstances I should prefer to die immediately, I should certainly answer yes.'[16]

Not only might this comment be described as insensitive, it points to the fallacy of believing that we can take our own life experiences and translate them into someone else's reality. The child born with Down's Syndrome will never have known anything else and cannot blindly be presumed to have an unacceptable quality of life simply because we know what we would lose if our situation changed.

For some, therefore, this very real difficulty is yet a further reason to prioritise the presumption in favour of life — in favour of treatment. Smith puts it this way:

> The fact that life is a *sine qua non* for the exercise of virtually all other rights, and that death is an irreversible event, contribute to the preservation of life assumption. When the life of a child or incompetent person is involved there is a particularly strong presumption in favour of preserving life. These are the weakest members of society and the least able to protect themselves. Therefore, society has a special obligation to protect the lives of children.[17]

These are fine words, but they do not in fact accurately describe the way in which the sanctity of life argument is applied. An absolute commitment to the sanctity of all life is absent in every community. Whether through laws about self-defence, engagement in war, the imposition of the death penalty or our failure to save every life that could be saved, we already concede that lives may be balanced and that some will be lost. Moreover, there are more subtle arguments in the clinical context which are adduced to dilute the commitment to preserving all lives. These range from the principle of double effect, that is, that it is permissable to shorten life if the intention is the alleviation of pain[18] through to the distinction between ordinary and extraordinary treatment. Even those most wedded to the sanctity of life, therefore, will also use theories — which for many are disingenuous — to facilitate abandonment of the principle pure and simple — to modify it in some significant ways.

For this reason, many are dissatisfied with the use of this principle as the primary basis for decision making and some believe that it is both reasonable and desirable that we do make decisions based on what the future seems likely to hold for the child itself. While acknowledging that the phrase 'quality of life' has 'unfortunate and misleading connotations',[19] Rhoden still believes that it has value. As she says,

> we have entered a new era, one where life in virtually any condition can be sustained, and where our massive medical technology can be misused by being overused. At even the most fundamental level, where we agree that an unconscious life need not be prolonged, a quality of life judgement is being made. Only when we recognise that such judgements are appropriate, lawful, and indeed inevitable can we discard the euphemisms that disguise them and the arbitrary dividing lines that oversimplify them. Then, and only then, can we face the challenge of drawing lines that protect the vast majority of disabled infants who can live lengthy, happy lives, but that allow non-treatment of those who cannot.[20]

Other commentators take a different approach. The utilitarian, for example, would feel no real need to consider quality of life as central. In the interests of maximising happiness, this approach would take account of a wider range of considerations than that of the individual child.[21] In this philosophy, in any event, the infant cannot be seen as the bearer of all human rights. The fact of birth does not make the baby a person, rather it makes it a potential person — in much the same way as a foetus or an embryo. As Kuhse and Singer have said, 'The infant and the child are physically the same organism, but the child is a *person* in the full sense of the term, and a newborn infant is not.'[22]

The logic of this position, according to them, is that 'the loss of life for newly born infants is, other things being equal, much less significant than the loss of life for an older child or adult.'[23] Glover would also point to the view that babies, not having rights in his philosophy, are effectively replaceable, and that the failure to maintain an infant with disability may be both in the interests of the parents, who will not have to cope with a disabled child, and in the wider interest, in that these same parents may be encouraged to have further healthy children.[24]

There is also one further approach taken, generally by those who do not subscribe to the view that children, once born, have a right to life no matter their physical or mental condition. This takes the form of pointing to the fact that infanticide is a feature of Western societies. Historically, it is claimed, selective decisions about which infant should live and which should die have been taken throughout the centuries. Modern medicine may have made them more acute, but they are not foreign to us. In other words, history would show that the tenacious repetition of our belief in the sanctity of life is a reflection of rhetoric rather than reality. However, Post suggests that this is merely a device used to bring 'the practice of infanticide into the moral mainstream'[25] and concludes that those who use it 'overstate the extent to which infanticide has occurred in Western history. The result is a fixed ideological litany of particular sources that is both selective and misrepresentative of history.'[26]

The battle for the moral high ground in these cases is clearly hard fought, even if it is seldom won. Yet one thing is absolutely clear, and that is that some infants will not be treated even when their lives could be saved. The prospect of their future life is seen as being so 'demonstrably awful'[27] that they will be allowed to die. This is not the place for a discussion as to whether or not it is morally better (or different) to kill rather than to let die in such situations, although this question will be considered later. Rather, it is a reflection of the reality of the moral maze into which infants with disability and their treatment throw us. Doubtless, it was simpler when babies with severe disability had no prospect of remaining alive. No ethical code was needed to reach conclusions — ultimately, nature decided for us. But this is no longer the case, and 'The non-treatment of newborn infants raises profound questions about life and death, about parental autonomy, and about medical decision-making'.[28] It also begs the question of what role the law might have.

Like it or not, decisions are made on a daily basis that some infants should not be kept alive. No one school of thought seems to have convinced parents, doctors or the law. The result is uncertainty, inconsistency and confusion. But even if we can find no overwhelmingly convincing ethical code that points to a definite conclusion on this most vexing of issues, there are further values which we might wish to see imposed on to the current picture. Perhaps most importantly, this might be achieved by addressing the question of who is the appropriate decision maker.

There are five possible sources of authority — doctors, parents, a combination of these, ethics committees and the law. It has already been said that doctors traditionally took the lead in these matters. Clinicians are not living in a vacuum and they may feel that their duties include the shouldering of this responsibility. Smith notes, 'Some physicians make the decision not to treat an infant without even consulting the parents. This is done, apparently, to avoid forcing the parents to make extremely difficult decisions, and perhaps in some cases, when the physician opposes treatment he believes the parent will demand.'[29] Decisions about whether or not a child should live may, therefore, be taken on the basis of the doctor's own bias, with no external scrutiny and no accountability. Moreover, the doctor may be driven by a feeling of failure. Presiding over a pregnancy and birth which results in a severely disabled infant may represent professional catastrophe to the doctor who is trained to produce only positive results.

It has been suggested, however, that the role of the doctor in such decisions is problematic. Not only will the physician likely depend on his or her own intuitions in reaching a decision, but, according to Robertson, failure to treat 'represents the only large-scale instance of involuntary euthanasia now being practised by the medical profession, at a time when most physicians and the public retain strong opposition to involuntary euthanasia in other circumstances'.[30]

But there is an additional problem associated with leaving such decisions in the hands of clinicians. As has been pointed out in earlier chapters, when something is characterised as being within the clinical judgement of the doctor, different tests are applied when the decisions are challenged. Subsuming an ethical dilemma within the medical model may be a common way of diverting attention from the complexities of what is going on, but it is none the less unsatisfactory. What is actually happening, like it or not, when doctors take these decisions is that they are choosing death over life for someone else. Clinical indications may well have a relevance in treatment decisions, but they should not be permitted to dominate when there is so much unease about such choices being made in the first place and so much at stake.

But if the decision is one for the doctor, then he or she will be

judged — in most jurisdictions — not on the inherent morality
of the outcome but on whether or not the choice was one which
fellow professionals regard as appropriate in the circumstances.
But it is already clear that:

> To view the doctor's duty to his patient as one which can be
> entirely explained by his fellow professionals may be an under-
> standable approach in some ways, but it none the less disguises
> two potentially important factors. First it makes the assump-
> tion that the nature and extent of the doctor's duty to his patient
> is solely definable in terms of those duties which are claimed
> to exist by the doctor and his colleagues ... Secondly, ... *ex
> hypothesi* it fails to take account of the actual intention of the
> doctor, by inferring his intention from the fact that behaviour
> of this type is professionally acceptable.[31]

In other words, when doctors make decisions, they are seldom
subject to the kind of rigorous scrutiny which would otherwise
apply. In Australasia, for example, Blank notes that although
parents have been successfully prosecuted for causing the death
of their children by failing to provide necessary medical treatment,
'there are no known instances where a health care professional
has been prosecuted'.[32] And this is so despite the strong words
of the court in the Australian case of *Re F*,[33] where the judge said,
'No parent, no doctor, no court has any power to determine that
the life of any child, however disabled that child may be, will be
deliberately taken from it .... [The law] does not permit decisions
to be made concerning the quality of life, nor does it enable any
assessment to be made as to the value of any human being.'[34]

Equally, the presumption that doctors always act beneficently
is one which, while we may be comfortable with it, cannot invariably be sustained. The doctor, perhaps because of his/her special

expertise, may be even less sanguine about the prospects of a child with disability than others, or, in fear of legal reprisals may be inclined to manage cases aggressively. Yet, despite the fact that the law claims to make no distinction between infants on the basis of their disability or lack of it, medical and legal practice tell us a different story. This was made clear in the UK case of *R* v. *Arthur*.[35] In this case, the doctor admitted that he had administered a powerful sedative to a child born suffering from Down's syndrome whose parents had rejected it, and had decided against offering the child nutrition and hydration. For technical reasons which are unimportant the charge against Dr Arthur was reduced from murder to attempted murder. What is important about the case is the final verdict. Despite an admission that the doctor's behaviour was intended to cause the infant's death, the judge instructed the jury in terms which clearly incorporated precisely the fears which have been expressed above. Given evidence that selective non-treatment was not uncommonly practised, and without even attempting an analysis of motivation, Farquharson, J. charged the jury in this way: 'I imagine that you will think long and hard before concluding that eminent doctors have evolved standards that amount to committing a crime.'[36] The jury did, and Dr Arthur was acquitted.

Public awareness that such decisions are being taken may however have led to a shift away from the presumption that doctors are always the best people to decide. Ellis comments that

> Physicians, formerly important decision makers in this area, may no longer play as prominent a role. To be sure, the physician must supply information to the appropriate decision maker concerning the infant's condition, prognosis with or without treatment, and the character and risks of treatment. But this special knowledge and expertise do not

give physicians the moral or legal authority to make life or death decisions for defective newborns.[37]

But if doctors are no longer deemed the appropriate holders of the relevant authority, then who is to supplant them? One very obvious answer might be the parents. After all, they are intimately connected to the situation and will *prima facie* shoulder the responsibility for caring for any child which is permitted or assisted to survive. For Kuhse and Singer this is convincing. In their view, 'it cannot be right for others to override the desire of parents that their severely disabled infant should be allowed to die, and then return that infant to the unwilling parents with all the consequences that bringing up such a child may have for them and their other children'.[38] Of course, this presumes that returning the child to the parents is the only option, which is not necessarily the case. However, it also assumes that disruption in the family is of equal moral weight to the right of the child to receive life-sustaining treatment, an assumption with which many would be uncomfortable.

Yet there is a strong lobby in favour of permitting parents to make these decisions. Phillips, for example, argues that:

Since the family must live with the consequence of any decision made with regard to sustaining or withholding treatment, it is imperative that the decision is ultimately left to the parents. Neither physicians, hospital infant care review committees, nor the legal system should be permitted to usurp the fundamental right that abides in parents to make important decisions with regard to what is best for the children they have brought into existence.[39]

Doubtless, parents are most intimately concerned with their own children, but this does not impute moral authority to decide that they should die because of their disability. The assertion that parents do have such authority is the result of a twofold phenomenon. The first part relates to a misconception of precisely what rights parents have over their children. Certainly, they are given (diminishing) rights in certain areas and they undoubtedly shoulder responsibilities in respect of their children. But these rights and responsibilities are not absolute or unchallengeable. As was said in the US case of *Prince* v. *Massachusetts*,[40] 'parents may be free to become martyrs themselves. But it does not follow that they are free, in identical circumstances, to make martyrs of their children'.[41]

The second strand is perhaps most strongly evident in the United States where the concept of family privacy has gained considerable ground. But even here, the liberty of parents to make decisions for their children is not taken to imply absolute and total discretion. In the case of *Wisconsin* v. *Yoder*,[42] for example, it was said that parental rights could be limited when 'parental decisions will jeopardise the health or safety of the child,'[43] and Smith identifies 'a modern trend towards increasing state review of, and interference with, parental decision making for children when those decisions may significantly harm the child'.[44] In the UK a similar point was made by Templeman, L. J. when he said that 'while great weight ought to be given to the views of the parents they are not views which necessarily must prevail'.[45]

It is important, therefore, that we do not confuse parental rights and responsibilities with *carte blanche* to make any decision whatsoever. Parents have had their views ignored in many cases where their behaviour would harm their children, even when their choice was based on other protected rights such as freedom of religious conviction. Nor does the fact that the decision to allow a child to die is generally taken on medical grounds differentiate it from other decisions, such as not to feed the child or to obtain medical treatment, both of which would — outside the clinical setting — amount to specific crimes. Finally, it cannot be assumed that parents will, any more than doctors, act in an entirely disinterested manner. Not only may they be sufficiently distressed to lack clarity of thought, but they may also be as concerned about their own future as that of their child. The family unit is not exempt from selfish motivation.

Neither doctors nor parents, then, can necessarily be said to be the best or most appropriate decision makers. Each carries their own prejudices and emotional baggage which may obscure principled assessment of the situation. Nonetheless, each is a key participant in the tragedy which is unfolding. Might it not, therefore, be argued that — despite the obvious shortcomings of each when viewed separately — in combination they may achieve the best outcome? Certainly, this is the preferred solution in some countries. In one Australian case, for example, it was said that, 'the accepted Australian standard is to leave decisions relating to the management of children with gross congenital malformation to be taken by parents and physicians together'.[46]

Indeed, it is probably the case that the parental/medical axis is the one which most frequently does make the choice. Robertson, for example, says that, 'it is now common practice for parents to request, and for physicians to agree, not to treat such infants'.[47] That this is so seems to reflect a congruence of views in many cases. While the doctor may not necessarily initiate the decision, his or her advice will doubtless help to shape the parental conclusion. The involvement of the parent in this conclusion will, therefore, be permissive. However, as Robertson continues, 'Whatever the morality of the ultimate choice, it seems unfair to subject the life of a helpless infant to the unguided discretion of parent and physician, particularly when they may have conflicting interests.'[48]

In any event, it is worth pausing at this point to take stock. All of the debate so far has suggested that there **are** competent decision makers here, but this conclusion might be changed if we extrapolate a little. What is common to the argument is that it focuses on specific kinds of children. The real test might be to ask whether or not we would feel the same way were the children in question not disabled. In other words, would we be happy to allow doctors and/or parents to decide that treatment to save life should be denied if it were not a child with disability? The only plausible answer to this question must be no. What underlies the choices made is not the issue of parental rights or clinical management, but is **in fact** a reflection of our attitudes to handicap. Raphael puts it bluntly:

> If we are honest with ourselves, the main argument for allowing a Down's syndrome baby to die is not that his life will be too much of a burden to him but that it will be too much of a burden to his immediate family; and if we judge that the child's right to life outweighs the burden to others of looking after him, there is very little reason to say that his right implies a burdensome duty for his parents and siblings rather than a duty for the community as a whole.[49]

These choices then are neither disinterested nor private. Shrouding them in medical jargon or familial privacy obfuscates, but does not reduce, the fact that as societies we have a responsibility for the vulnerable and that it is on our shoulders that the burden must ultimately rest. If we do not provide adequate alternatives for families who cannot cope with a child with disability, we condemn it to die. If a right to life depends on perfection, then clinical evidence could lead to rejection of those who cannot meet such an exacting standard. In any event, the combination of parents and clinicians does not address the fundamental issues any more satisfactorily than does the option of either of them acting individually.

It seems clear, therefore, that analysis of these parties as decision-makers does not necessarily lead to the kind of openness, consistency and moral tone of decision making which I suggested earlier were of vital importance. Decision making with such grave consequences is not the prerogative of any individual or group merely because they happen to be involved in a certain way, nor because they are physically present when decisions have to be taken. But, assuming that these decisions will be made, is there any alternative? It is emotionally appealing to think that the outcome will be determined by those who, because of nature or professional standards, might seem to have the most to gain or lose, but it may actually be that this very fact is sufficient to justify their disenfranchisement if what we seek is the application of fair principles and an equitable allocation of care.

In the United States, there is a contemporary trend towards using ethics committees as fora for tackling sensitive and complex issues. Although in other countries their role is often limited to judging the ethics of research, they may provide a way forward. After a shaky start (in the UK at least) ethics committees are gaining favour as decision-making bodies, not least because they are bound to represent views from professionals and lay people. This is not the place to indulge in debate about their actual effectiveness, although it is and has been a matter of some concern. Nonetheless, as an alternative to the self-interested decisions which might be made by the others, they do have one obvious advantage in that they may serve to distance the decision from those whose emotions and self-concern may dominate.

If it is, as Smith says, 'unacceptable to withhold life-saving treatment from an infant because the child will have a negative effect on the family, the medical community, or others',[50] then might not independent ethical review committees provide just the bridge necessary to ensure that the considerations which are taken into account are the appropriate ones? The answer to this depends, of course, on what values we seek to endorse. For some, the committee based decision would be an intrusion into the rights of doctors and parents. Phillips, for example, says, 'A committee comprised of members having no real personal or moral stake in the outcome of the decision whether to sustain or with-hold treatment must not be permitted to take the place of parents in making decisions regarding their own children'.[51]

For others, it is a system with proven inconsistencies and lacking the procedural regularities which decisions of this sort demand. Thus, if procedural fairness and formal justice are to inform our approach to infants with disability, then arguably decision by committee is no better than decision by doctor or parent. The content of the decision may be less emotional, but ultimately it remains an *ad hoc* decision, and will be likely to be influenced by just as many unstated assumptions as those of other possible decision makers.

Despite this caveat, Rhoden would endorse the use of committees in this area. She believes that 'ethical committees are a good procedural safeguard. They respect the family's role and do not seek to displace parental autonomy ... '[52] For some, of course, this might be a further reason to **discourage** decision by committee, since it suggests that they work at their best, in her terms at least, when they effectively retransfer authority to the family, or at least give considerable weight to the family's views. The critical point, however, is one which she also makes. 'Although ethics committees cannot eliminate uncertainties or occasional errors, if they work from clearly articulated principles and guidelines they can promote consistency in these cases and prevent potential abuses without simultaneously eroding the authority of the family'.[53]

Parents and doctors may feel that they are best suited to making these decisions. Others, however, would argue that never is the role of the law more important than in such cases. Indeed, Rhoden has effectively conceded this point, since her ideal ethical committee would be one which articulates and depends on the kinds of standards for which we traditionally look to the law. Of course, we need to know just what it is that we expect the law to achieve, but for Robertson:

> A minimum requirement should guarantee certainty of rule and rule enforcement, thereby informing people of the limits of their discretion and enhancing freedom by permitting them to take legal rules into account. In addition to certainty, however, the law should create a system of expectations that resolves conflicting interests consistent with prevailing morality and our sense of what is just and right.[54]

Yet for many years, law was rarely, if ever, involved in these decisions. Even now, it is likely that legal standards will be brought into the fray only where a dispute exists about the rightness of a proposed piece of behaviour. Certainly, there are arguments against legal involvement, whether in the form of courts or in the form of legislation. Law is often taken to be a blunt instrument when matters of such sensitivity arise. But this is to mistake the actual value of the law which lies in its principles more than its structural manifestation. Doubtless, many will find resonance in Phillips's view that, 'Judges should not be held to hold the answers to all questions, especially those in which they have considerably less expertise or interest than those who will be deeply and eternally affected by the resolution of the dispute.'[55] However, closer inspection shows that there are flaws in this analysis.

For Phillips the critical determinants of the 'right' decision hinge on the nature of the parental interest in the child and the possession of medical expertise. But it has been suggested here that, although these may be useful in informing decisions, they are by no means the only considerations which are of relevance. Bigger societal concerns must also play a part, and stringently applied standards must be observed if lives are to be deliberately lost. Campbell and Duff admit that, outside a legal framework, 'Bad decisions are possible...'[56] but conclude that 'many safeguards against bad choices are already in existence and it can be argued that the courts are unlikely to be any better in dealing with these enormously complex problems'.[57] And Whitelaw contends that, 'In cases where thorough medical investigation and lengthy discussion have led the medical team and the parents to choose withdrawal of treatment, there seems little benefit in involving legal procedures'.[58]

The question to be asked, however, is benefit for whom? Undoubtedly, parents and doctors will not have taken their decision lightly and they may well regard legal intervention as inappropriate, are we striving trying to respect these decisions or to protect children from overly emotional or clinically doom-laden assessments? There may be no benefit to be derived by doctors and parents from legal involvement, but there may well be for the child.

Law, whether statutory or common, undoubtedly has the capacity to balance interests and to work from principle. But for many, the adversarial nature of the court setting is a drawback when dealing with sensitive issues. Certainly, this was the view in the US case of *Satz* v. *Perlmutter*,[59] and, it is also a view held by a number of judges in the UK. However, as shown in the previous chapter, it may well be that this assertion is flawed by the assumptions on which it is based. Where the outcome of any decision is of such gravity as the deprivation of the capacity to reproduce or the denial of life-preserving treatment, there may in fact be an even stronger case for the questions to be tested in an adversarial way, with someone independently representing the interests of the individual whose rights are under threat. Whether or not judges always get it right may be less relevant than the fact that the proposed course of action has been rigorously scrutinised and thoroughly tested. As Robertson said, 'In resolving the emotional and ethical dilemmas that confront parents of defective infants, it is surprising that law and legal values have rarely been invoked. The law's long experience with protecting minority rights and its concern with procedure and decision-making processes may offer a path out of this troublesome thicket.'[60]

But if the courts are to achieve this, then, as always, it is vital that they operate to principles and tests which are suited to the issue under consideration. Clearly, this throws us back on to the problem of just what tests can appropriately be used. As usual, there seem to be two — substituted judgement and 'best interests'. It is not necessary to restate at length what the problems are with these tests, but it should be obvious that a substituted judgement test is peculiarly unsuited to decisions regarding neonates with disability since, more than ever, they could only be based on guesswork and would doubtless import the prejudices which the decision maker might have.

In any event, the tradition of the courts in cases involving welfare is to prefer the 'best interests' test, and it is the test most commonly applied in these situations. The fact that it is commonly used, however, does not necessarily mean that it is unproblematic. The problems of this test are perhaps particularly acute when end of life decisions are being made. As Raphael has said, 'I always find it difficult to interpret the idea that death can be the interest or the best interest of someone. Since death will terminate his existence, how can one speak of there being any interests, positive or negative, arising from death?'[61] Of course, one answer could be that, since we allow adults to choose to die rather than to suffer, by endorsing their competent refusal of life saving treatment, then this should not be denied to those who, by reason of lack of competence, cannot make that decision for themselves.

However, this response would not adequately deal with Raphael's point. The reason that we endorse these competent decisions is not a recognition that it is in someone's best interests to die, but is rather the result of respect for their autonomous choice. Perhaps a better way to look at the question is to refine the 'best interests' test to encapsulate the notion of benefit. If we ask, will treatment benefit someone, then we ask a different question. As Rhoden says:

> The principle of nonmaleficence…requires that the harm of a proposed treatment be outweighed by a countervailing benefit. Benefit, in turn, must be defined in terms of the whole person, and not merely in terms of isolated organ systems or purely biological responses: to be benefited, a patient must have the potential for partaking in some of those experiences that make life characteristically human.[62]

Looked at from this perspective, then, it should be feasible that some decisions not to treat could be made. However, Rhoden's warning that we should look at the totality of the outcome of treatment is still, by itself, insufficient to ensure that decisions are not made based either on individual prejudice or over-emphasis on clinical recommendations. Although traditions vary, it is clear that, in the UK at least, at present courts 'allow themselves to be led by the medical profession'.[63] As Wells, says, given that this is the case, 'it is not surprising that ... [they] appear to pay lip service to the sanctity of life while leaving a vast discretion to the doctor in charge in consultation with parents'.[64]

For these reasons, there is an increasing trend in some countries toward legislative rather than judicial controls. In the US there is a considerable amount of legislation bearing directly on such cases, ranging from child abuse regulations to The Emergency Medical Treatment and Active Labour Act. The recent case of *Baby K*[65] shows the extent to which legislation is in itself problematic. In this case, the mother's demand for treatment which doctors would probably regard as futile, if not cruel, was validated by legislation which was actually designed to fill the gaps in health care provision which shame the US health care system. In reality, the legislation which she used was not directly designed to deal with the kind of situation in which she and her child found themselves and this too is one reason why the law may seem to be the wrong mechanism to be used.

Yet a legislative response which is directly concerned with the situation under review may reflect the values which, this discussion has suggested, are critical to the appropriate, consistent and compassionate resolution of these different cases. By drawing the line narrowly, and by requiring that decisions are tested in an appropriate forum, we may simultaneously reduce the opportunity for abuse and yet still permit some babies to die. Perhaps even more vitally, the law has the capacity to attain fairness and consistency in decision making. Although Phillips would argue that these decisions should not be delegated 'to a legislature that has neither the time, the expertise, nor the interest to make such important life and death decisions ...'[66] this criticism is ill-founded.

The point is that, unless the lives of children with disability are to be subject to the emotional decisions of parents or the clinical predictions of doctors, the 'expertise' that is necessary is the expertise of independence; not clinical expertise, nor even a claimed expertise in parenting. It is the independence of the law which commends its use in these cases. By superimposing legislative guidelines on the judiciary, we have the potential to double the impact of principles that derive from the law's tradition and its capacity to take account of new dilemmas.

Of course, for some, there will never be a justification for allowing infants with disability to die. Their objection will be based on considerations ranging from a belief in the sanctity of all life to the discrimination which seems inherent in selective decisions of this sort. The former objection is essentially unmeetable, since we either believe in it or we don't, but the latter can be substantially met by laws which recognise this as a genuine fear and are framed accordingly. Starting from Smith's premise that the state 'must protect the children who are born with a severe disability',[67] and based on criteria which Robertson writes 'represent a collective social judgement, rather than idiosyncratic choices of parents and committees, as to when social costs outweigh individual benefits ...'[68] legislation coupled with judicial review may provide maximum protection of the vulnerable infant.

Inevitably, there will remain those, like Phillips, who believe that 'There are some areas into which the law should not tread. Medical treatment for seriously ill newborns is one such area'.[69] But these will be commentators who regard the decisions being taken as solely personal and/or clinical. Medicine may well have created or exacerbated the problems faced in the paediatric wards, but the resolution of these problems requires assessments which transcend the clinical. Certainly, courts will wish to take account of parental views and clinical prognoses, but these cannot be treated as definitive. The issues involved are too significant to be left to partial decision making, however well intentioned.

In conclusion, then, it can be said that the case of newborns with disability exposes most clearly the dilemmas which medical advance can pose. These are dilemmas for all of us and not simply for the doctors or for the unfortunate parents. The progress made in medicine is in itself to be welcomed, but yet again we would be unwise to treat the question as one which can be primarily resolved medically. In addition, it can be said that — at least in some countries — the courts have to date shown themselves still to be in thrall to the medical/parental axis. Even in those countries which have attempted legislative intervention, the apparent failure of other laws to offer rigorous protection coupled with compassion show that we must re-evaluate the principles on which life and death decisions can or should be made. Only revision of legislative requirements tempered with sensitive, but adversarial, trial of the facts will satisfy the values and principles which must be elucidated and applied in these most vexing of situations.

7 Choosing Life or Death

The face of death and dying has changed dramatically in recent years. From being an essentially private event or process, it has become the focus of public interest. From being a process whose path is unstoppable, it has become subject to the increasing capacity of medicine to intervene and postpone the ultimate outcome. These changes have resulted from two main sources. First, many more people will now die in health-care institutions than at home. Second, medical advance and technology can result in prolonging life or slowing the dying process. Even where cure is not possible, drugs and other therapies may offer life-extension.

These factors have combined to result in what Capron calls 'the medicalisation of death'.[1] The tendency to medicalise sensitive and difficult decisions is no less clear in this situation than it has been in the other chapters in this book. Yet our attitudes to death are vital to the way in which we live. As Illich says, 'A society's image of death reveals the level of independence of its people, their personal relatedness, self-reliance, and aliveness.'[2]

Advances in medicine are generally perceived to be good. Certainly, they may result in the restoration to health of those who would otherwise die. But they may also have a less positive side. The capacity to sustain existence brings into sharp focus the question of whether or not all life should be preserved, and the fact that alleviation of symptoms or cure may now be possible may result in the return of paternalism. Medical advance, therefore, may affect end of life considerations in both a positive and a negative way.

Just as 'medicine seems to be sharpening its tools to do battle with death itself, treating death as if it were just one more disease',[3] an increasingly rights conscious society has begun to demand the right to deal with death on its own terms. The movement for choice in end of life matters is growing exponentially, and evidence from around the world shows increasing numbers of individuals seeking to control their own death and increasing numbers of doctors prepared to abide by such decisions.[4] No longer is it advisable to adopt the simplistic view that what we can do we should do. The dilemmas posed by accepting this are both generated by and affect medicine. As Kass says, 'medicine, as well as the community that supports it, appears to be perplexed regarding its purpose .... When its powers were fewer, its purpose was clearer.'[5]

However, even if it is agreed that medical practitioners are conceding the increasing complexity of their role at the end of a patient's life, the power of medicine is not diminished. To a large extent the role of medicine is absolutely central to the 'degree of lived freedom'[6] experienced by individuals in this, as in other, situations. While medicine may sometimes be accused of concentrating on the technical, the public is increasingly concerned about quality of life. A 1987 report showed that 'the new powers of medicine have proved to be a mixed blessing. Our capacity to prolong life in many cases exceeds our capacity to restore health.'[7]

Death and dying are, of course, surrounded by powerful taboos. Most countries, whatever their history, continue to proclaim the sanctity of life as a primary value. Even in those societies where exceptions are made, for example where the death penalty is legal, the rhetoric of the sanctity of life has immense symbolic power. Thus, taboos have built up around suicide, assisted death and euthanasia which are sustained not by the wishes of the individual but rather by the repetition of this dogmatic position.

Equally, however, medicine has shown itself capable of maintaining existence for those who may remain alive without the capacity to experience life or to ask for its termination. The dilemmas posed here are perhaps the most acute, and point to the difficulty of balancing interests. Adherence to the sanctity of life will result in moral confusion. If all life is sacred then those who are technically alive must be shown equal respect for their life, even if, as Kass puts it, this results in long periods of time 'kept company by cardiac pacemakers and defibrillators, respirators, aspirators, oxygenators, catheters, and his intravenous drip. Ties to the community of men are replaced by attachments to an assemblage of machines.'[8]

The fundamental taboos which surround the very subject of death permit the perpetuation of an approach to it which may have a number of consequences. First, those who actively choose death may be regarded as irrational or lacking in legal competence. This is particularly so when medicine can offer hope of a cure or palliation of symptoms. Capron accuses the courts in the United States of using concepts such as '"incompetency" as a way of overriding patient decisions they consider unreasonable',[9] even though the general rule of law (expressed here in an English judgement) is that '[a] decision to refuse medical treatment by a patient capable of making the decision does not have to be sensible, rational or well-considered'.[10]

Second, some individuals may be so afraid of a life without prolonged quality that they choose suicide as an option. Angell, for example, has noted that: 'The very high suicide rate in older Americans is due partly to concern that they will be unable to stop treatment if hospitalised …. Some people now fear living more than dying, because they dread becoming prisoners of technology.'[11]

If this is so, then the sanctity of life principle will have the paradoxical effect of adding to rather than reducing avoidable deaths.

Third, societies may be faced with an increasing demand for legal reform to permit active assistance in choosing the timing and manner of the individual's own death. Recent reforms in the state of Oregon, The Netherlands and the Northern Territory in Australia[12] are in the vanguard of a radical rethinking of societal views on assisted death and euthanasia, even although those states which tolerate or authorise some kind of assistance in dying still represent a small minority of countries.

Finally, medical advances require resolution of the question of what is to be done in respect of the person who is incompetent, with no hope of recovery and with no clear advance expression of wishes. Strict adherence to the principle of the sanctity of life results in such individuals being maintained in an insentient form for what, in some cases, may be a very long time. Without clear justifications for the termination of treatment, life which has no quality for the person living it will be prolonged merely because the technology to do so exists. As Annas says:

> Although states no longer have the legal authority to make slaves of people, they now do have authority to permit medical technology disconnected from any medical purpose to make slaves of incompetent citizens. Medical technologies have taken on a life of their own and seem to have been ceded more rights to be used than previously competent patients have rights to have their families make decisions about such use on their behalf.[13]

Thus, the uses of medical advances and technologies have opened up a wide-ranging debate, and one which is not yet resolved. For some, the central consideration will relate to what they are permitted to decide for themselves. For others, the issue of major importance will be what they have to decide on behalf of others and whether or not their decision is lawful. Demographic change means that increasingly decisions will have to be made by others about the health care of, for example, elderly relatives. Shepard claims, for example, that 'Most Americans eventually find themselves called upon to make some kind of medical decisions for parents or grandparents. The advance of medical technology and the concomitant opportunity for prolonging life have made these occasions more numerous, but they are hardly new to the 1990s.'[14] And Weir notes further that '[t]he American Hospital Association estimates that many of the six thousand daily deaths in the United States are orchestrated by patients, relatives, and physicians'.[15]

What is new, however, is the way in which decisions about the end of life have become the object of public scrutiny. This has come about for different reasons. On the one hand, it is clear that the contemporary way of death is anathema to some people, resulting as it may in a death without dignity. On the other hand, concern that life will be judged by others and found wanting has raised concerns in its own right. As Capron puts it: 'I never want to have to wonder whether the physician coming into my hospital room is wearing the white coat (or the green scrubs) of a healer … or the black hood of the executioner.'[16]

It would be foolish to imply that, because of the dilemmas raised by medicine's capacities, medicine is somehow in the wrong. Medical advances have restored many to health and saved many lives which even a short time ago would have been needlessly lost. However, as with all medical advances, their impact is not value free. In this area, as in others, medicine affects our lives in ways which are subtle and complex. Of fundamental significance, then, is how that impact is controlled and the extent to which it is pervasive.

Most obviously, and doubtless entirely innocently, medicine presents us with the initial dilemma. If medicine were less efficient, then decisions of this sort would not be made at all. People would face death in the traditional manner. Medicine's capacities to alleviate the pain which is associated with many deaths, to prolong existence in some cases and to provide a compassionate and caring service are not in doubt. However, the unfortunate converse of this is also true in some cases. For some, the nature of dying will involve considerable suffering. For others, life will be maintained, but in a state of mere existence. As Capron makes clear, medical advance means that 'There is no such thing as a "natural" death. Somewhere along the way for just about every patient, death is forestalled by human choice and human action, or death is allowed to occur because of human choice.'[17]

Even if some individuals prefer to let nature take its course, then, the reality is that decisions are being made on behalf of other people all the time. The question is, who is making these decisions and on what basis? As the last chapter shows, there is a paradox in the legal systems of most developed countries in that decisions taken by third parties which lead to death, without being able to ascertain the wishes of the person whose life it is, may be endorsed by our law, while competent decisions made by the individual in question are generally given no legal standing.

Doubtless, some would simply say that decisions of this sort should never be taken, but the reality is that they are, and for many it is right that the concept of choice should be applied to dying as much as it is to living. Evidence from around the world shows that the combination of medical capabilities and the rights-consciousness of communities has resulted in many deaths being 'chosen' in one way or another. As Kuhse says:

the question is not *whether* decisions to end human lives

ought to be made but, rather, *who* makes these decisions, and on the basis of what principles or values. For the fact is that such decisions are already being made, and inevitably must be made, in modern hospitals.[18]

The question of who makes these decisions is one which is rightly the interest of the community as a whole, and perhaps inevitably, therefore, the interest of the law. This was not always so, and for some the fact that clinicians were prepared to take decisions on their own and without external scrutiny was a 'great advantage'[19] to society. For others, to invest one group with such powers was unthinkable. However, whatever was done in the past, a series of cases over the last few decades has shown that increasingly courts are becoming involved in scrutinising the basis of decision making and judging its lawfulness. As Lord Mustill put it in the (UK) case of *Airedale NHS Trust* v. *Bland*, 'the authority of the state, through the medium of the courts, is being invoked to permit one group of its citizens [doctors] to terminate the life of another'.[20]

In this tragic case, a young man who had been a victim of a disaster at a football ground had remained unconscious for several years. He was diagnosed as being in a condition known as persistent vegetative state (PVS). In this condition, he could have survived for many years with the assistance of nasogastric feeding and good nursing care, but he would never have regained consciousness. His doctor and his parents petitioned the court to allow for the withdrawal of the feeding mechanism so that he might be allowed to die. This authority was eventually given by the House of Lords.

The apparent shift of power from the doctor to the courts is one which probably rests on several factors. Undoubtedly, doctors are increasingly aware that they are vulnerable to the law, and it is reasonable to conclude, as Capron does, that 'in an era in which physicians and other health care providers feel themselves constantly under a siege of litigation, decisions for death are driven with increasing frequency into the courts.'[21]Equally, it is accepted that decisions of this sort are not definable solely as medical decisions. No matter the value of professional codes or professional agreement, they cannot and do not provide a sufficient explanation of the ethical questions which underpin decisions, nor can or should they be seen as necessarily able to provide an ethical answer.[22] For the individuals concerned the 'best' outcome will be one which reflects their own values, perhaps even irrespective of the medical recommendation. And, of course, the ability to 'choose' death raises new and important dilemmas of fundamental importance to society; dilemmas which transcend their clinical content.

Undoubtedly, therefore, the law has a role to play in setting the parameters within which choices can be made. This is undoubtedly an extremely difficult task, and one on which judges throughout the world have disagreed. Particular problems arise where the individual is incompetent, and it is here that the law is most often involved. Initial attention will, therefore, be focused on this group, and in particular the person who is in persistent vegetative state, since laws which may accommodate competent decision making are not available in such cases. Moreover, the way in which the law treats the incompetent lays bare the bases on which decisions are made.

While some courts have felt able to make decisions for incompetents, others have indicated that this a matter for the legislature. Still others, for example in the New Zealand case of *Auckland Area Health Board* v. *Attorney General*,[23] have indicated that:

the issues to which this kind of case gives rise cannot be resolved by strict logic, and certainly not by legal logic. In

the end questions will be best determined by the application of common principles of humanity and common sense.
Those principles are not outside the law, but nor are they
the prerogative of the law.[24]

Whatever the best framework for decision making may be, it is
certainly one which requires the independence of the law (whether
judge made or statutory) to test in an accountable and transpar-
ent manner what must surely be one of the most complex and
definitive conclusions which can be reached by any person. Yet,
analysis of case law would suggest that the very reason for turning to the law — namely its independence — may be defeated
ab initio. The medicalisation of death leads to an over-emphasis
in law on the ethics and the expertise of the doctor, and a subsequent under-representation of other value systems. Thus, what
the doctor knows, and what the doctor believes to be so, have
profoundly influenced the agenda which the courts set themselves
and the bases on which they reach conclusions.

In many countries, therefore, the paradigm within which decisions are made is necessarily situational or contextual. The
governing principles, the questions to be asked and the answers
provided will depend heavily on the clinical view of the issues,
the perceived constraints of medical ethics and what the doctor,
and his or her colleagues, believe to be the 'best' outcome.
However, '[s]urely much more than medical ethics is involved in
these decisions? The fact that they most often arise in a hospital
setting does not make them solely or even predominantly
medical.'[25]

Yet, in the New Zealand case referred to earlier, the court said:
'Generally speaking, the courts certainly will not wish to intrude
upon what they ... perceive to be the legitimate province of the
doctors and their patients. Undoubtedly, the courts will be slow

to respond to any invitation to resolve an issue which is essentially a clinical or medical decision.'[26]

When dealing with those who cannot speak for themselves, for example the patient in persistent vegetative state, the petition facing the courts will often come from a combination of relatives and doctors. In strict law, of course, relatives have no legal standing to make decisions on behalf of an adult, and most probably have only limited powers in respect of children — namely, to act in their best interests. But the courts too have an obligation to act in the best interests of the person concerned. The question is, how does the court conclude upon what best interests may be? On the answer to this question much hinges.

There are two main ways in which 'best interests' may be determined. The first applies a strict 'best interests' test in which an attempt is made to balance benefits and drawbacks. The second, more favoured in the United States, is to identify, by means of substituted judgement, what the person would have wanted had they been in a position to tell the court.[27] Although not traditionally described as a form of the 'best interests' test, the latter arguably is in fact just that. What differs is the kind of interests which are taken as important. The tendency in the strict test is to look most closely at the clinical considerations while the latter, which has found no favour in UK courts, addresses (however fancifully) a broader range of values which the person may have held. Thus, rather than looking at clinical outcome, the substituted judgement test takes the interests concerned to include previously expressed autonomous wishes. To this extent, it is significantly less influenced by medical considerations, and despite its obvious drawbacks it may more accurately reflect what the individual would have wanted, rather than simply relying on what the doctor thinks is best. Of course, a further problem is that, not only do decisions made on this basis represent mere speculation but as Capron puts it, 'just as technology makes death a matter of human choice, the transfer of this choice from the hospital room to the courtroom makes death a matter of *judicial* choice, or so the judge may well feel. Thus, once medicine is no longer the issue, the question becomes: What deaths will the state (through its duly constituted officers) allow?'[28]

However, no matter which test is used, the influence of medicine is evident. To an extent, this is inevitable, since — if the court is to exercise its judgement in respect of an incompetent person to permit a death to occur — then it will need to have regard to the clinical diagnosis and prognosis which triggered the perceived need for choice in the first place. Equally, the decision will only be required if medicine could prolong life but prefers not to. The agenda then is already set. Now, it might be thought that given the public protestations of adherence to the sanctity of all life, the answer would be straightforward. Indeed, it might have been expected that the question would never have been raised at all. However, this is manifestly not so, given the number of cases confronting courts.

It is here that we begin to see the inroads made into other values by the dependence of the law on medical evidence. From proclaiming a strict adherence to the sanctity of life, courts begin to distance themselves from the logical outcome of this and to protest, for example, that 'there is no absolute rule that the patient's life must be prolonged by ... treatment or care, if available, regardless of the circumstances'.[29] The circumstances to be taken into account are generally based on clinical evidence of potential outcome and '[t]he decision whether or not the continued treatment and care of a PVS patient confers any benefit on him is essentially one for the practitioners in charge of his case'.[30]

Of course, as an argument, this potentially fails on two counts. First, it hangs on the question of benefit or 'best interests', yet, as Lord Mustill pointed out in the Bland case, the very nature of the diagnosis of PVS means that the person doesn't have any interests to be considered.[31] Second, having made that leap of illogic, it then proceeds to permit clinicians to describe what these 'interests' are. In other words, the individual's fate is decided on the basis of entirely flawed reasoning, but reasoning which accords with what doctors regard as being within the ambit of medical ethics.

Having defined the issues at stake largely from the medical perspective it is then open to the courts to apply one further test — namely to ask, as a form of validation what other doctors would do in the same circumstances. This professional test is widely used in medical negligence cases where its application has been the subject of considerable criticism.[32] Its appropriateness to issues of life and death is surely even more open to debate unless the decision is seen as substantially, or exclusively, dependent on medicine.

Although some judges have expressed concern about the use of a professional test in these matters, the fact that the preliminary debate is couched in clinical terms has led others to apply it without apparent concern. This is shown most starkly in the case of patients in persistent vegetative state. If the underlying issue is medical, then it is necessary to encapsulate what is proposed within the medical model also. In the case of the PVS patient, life can be prolonged — sometimes for many years — by the relatively simple expedient of nasogastric feeding and good nursing care.

But if the individual is to die, then what is done to bring about that death must be something which is within the authority of the doctor to do. For some people, feeding and hydration are part of the basics of life — they are not medical matters. Indeed, it is clear that if a non-doctor had an incompetent person within their care and failed to provide nutrition and hydration they would face the full wrath of the law. It is here that the contextual nature of current legal analysis takes centre stage.

In the House of Lords, the difficulty posed by this conundrum was summarily swept aside by one judge who satisfied himself that the continuance or withdrawal of nasogastric feeding was appropriately judged by doctors, saying: 'There is overwhelming evidence that, in the medical profession, artificial feeding is regarded as a form of medical treatment; and even if it is not strictly medical treatment, it must form part of the medical care of the patient'.[33]

Thus, in his view — and that of other judges throughout the world — the fact that doctors regard something as medical treatment is sufficient to make it so. In two statements in 1986 and 1989, the American Medical Association endorsed this view.[34] Nutrition and hydration are in this model seen as equivalent to artificial ventilation, whose withdrawal is generally accepted when it is regarded as futile — in other words, when it cannot keep the person alive or serves no clinical function. Thus:

> doctors have a lawful excuse to discontinue ventilation when there is no medical justification for continuing that form of medical assistance. To require the administration of a life-support system when such a system has no further medical function or purpose and serves only to defer the death of the patient is to confound the purpose of medicine.[35]

Ignoring for the moment the question as to whether or not the 'purpose of medicine' (however that is defined) is the ultimate value to be served, this assertion imports somewhat disingenuously yet another contextual matter. By addressing the 'who' and not the 'why' it disguises the hard fact that the outcome will be a death. It is absolutely clear that the death is both foreseen and intended and would normally therefore amount to a criminal act. But, because it is a doctor who is involved, the law will treat the matter differently. This different treatment seems to rest on two central tenets. First that the doctor's actions will be intended to be beneficent and second that the doctor is in a unique situation because the issue has been defined as medical.

Manifestly, doctors will generally be taken — and rightly so — to be acting beneficently and not maliciously. However, this is never susceptible of proof, and in any event motive is irrelevant to the nature of a criminal act. I too may act beneficently in helping a loved one to die, but I would certainly be open to criminal charges. On the second point, Lord Goff in the Bland case, made what for him was a satisfactory distinction between the doctor and the 'interloper', saying 'the doctor's conduct is to be differentiated from that of, for example, an interloper who maliciously switches off a life support machine because, although the interloper may perform exactly the same act as the doctor who discontinues life support, his doing so constitutes interference with the life-prolonging treatment then being administered by the doctor.'[36]

It is surely clear at this stage that sophistry is being engaged in to ensure that the courts may hold the behaviour of a doctor to be lawful while at the same time criminalising exactly the same behaviour were it carried out by a third party. But there is still one further device which was then used to distinguish the withdrawal of nutrition and hydration by a doctor from its withdrawal by someone else. Lord Goff continued: 'whereas the doctor, in discontinuing life support, is simply allowing his patient to die of his pre-existing condition, the interloper is actively intervening to stop the doctor from prolonging the patient's life, and such conduct cannot possibly be categorised as an omission'.[37]

It is a core belief of many doctors that there is a critical difference between actively killing a patient and omitting to save them. In general law it is, of course the case, that we are culpable for our acts but not for our omissions. However, the doctor is in precisely the opposite position, since the existence of a pre-existing duty of care renders acts and omissions of equal culpability. Even assuming that the difference between an act and an omission where the outcome is both intended and foreseen is a real one (and many would dispute this) the fact that the doctor owes a duty of care renders this irrelevant in law. In any event, as Beauchamp and Childress point out:

> Nothing about killing or letting die entails judgements about actual wrongness or rightness, or about the beneficence or nonmaleficence of the action. Rightness and wrongness depend on the merit of the justification underlying the action, not on the type of action it is. Neither killing nor letting die, therefore, is *per se* wrongful, and in this regard they are to be distinguished from murder, which is *per se* wrong. Both killing and letting die are *prima facie* wrong, but can be justified under some circumstances. [38]

It is also worth noting at this point that the desire to distinguish between acts and omission may have one further consequence which is seldom remarked upon. The use of this distinction serves to focus the moral spotlight on the act. Commentators and judges alike are so bound up in their efforts to condemn active participation in the death of another, so in thrall to the alleged difference between acts and omissions, that they presuppose the morality of omissions. Yet, an omission too may be malicious, wilful, even criminal. The intellectual struggle needed to maintain that it is distinct from an act may serve to render us relatively more casual about endorsing an omission and/or to further emphasise its medical context as both a justification for it and a reason for approving it.

Thus, although this perceived distinction may be comfortable for doctors, and may satisfy some judges, it is at best disingenuous and at worst dangerous. As Rachels says, 'both the costs and benefits encourage us, selfishly, to view killing as worse than letting die. It is to our own advantage to believe this, and so we do.'[39] Not all judges, however, are comfortable with this approach. In the *Bland* case, Lord Mustill declared 'acute unease'[40] about using the acts/omissions doctrine as a way of resolving the problem, noting that 'however much the terminologies may differ, the ethical status of the two courses of action is for all relevant purposes indistinguishable'.[41] His concern was that the judgement in this case would 'emphasise the distortions of a legal structure which is already both morally and intellectually misshapen'.[42]

In addition, even if there were a difference between the two, the notion that the doctor's behaviour is merely 'letting die' and the behaviour of anyone else would be 'killing' is equally open to challenge. In the case of a person whose condition is terminal, removal or withdrawing of treatment no matter who it is undertaken by would allow the patient to die, or, in either case could be seen as an act of killing. The fact that one is a doctor does not alter the categorisation of the event in strict terms, even although courts have fallen into the trap of holding that it does. In any event, for the patient in PVS it is nonsensical to suggest that the patient dies of the pre-existing condition, no matter who removes the feeding.

The patient in PVS is not terminally ill. With appropriate care, he or she may survive for many years. Unarguably what causes the death of the patient is the removal of the feeding. Faced with the truth of this, courts have tried further tests to ensure that they are not seen as condoning euthanasia. Given that it has already been made clear that the sanctity of life is not a principle which is adhered to without exception, it might be thought that the euthanasia question would be relatively easily resolved.

We do not demand that people live — we tolerate suicide and attempted suicide, and we endorse the right of a competent patient to refuse life-saving treatment. In other words, we respect an autonomous decision even if we do not approve of it. If the condition of an individual facilitates a third party decision that life is not preferable to non-life, then surely the clearest evidence we could have of what it is ethical to do is where the individual him or herself actually says this clearly, repeatedly and unequivocally.

However, courts are reluctant to concede this, perhaps in part because they do not approve of euthanasia, but to a large extent because the guiding principles in these cases are those of **medical** ethics. This is not to say that some judges are unaware of the lack of logic of their position, nor that they have not addressed the outcome which flows from this approach. In the Bland case, for example, Lord Browne-Wilkinson, addressing the consequences of the decision to withdraw artificial feeding, asked this question; '[h]ow can it be lawful to allow a patient to die slowly, though painlessly, over a period of weeks from a lack of food but unlawful to produce his immediate death by a lethal injection'.[43] He was forced to conclude, 'I find it difficult to find a moral answer to that question'.[44]

Equally, if death is the desired outcome, and there is no difference between an act and an omission since, as McLean says, 'the doctor who withdraws treatment, or withholds it, is legally an active participant in the death … ',[45] then it might be agreed that it is 'obligatory to criticise a legal regimen which permits death where the individual has made no choice for it yet criminalises it where a competent decision has been made'.[46] As was noted in the case of *State of Georgia* v. *McAfee*,[47] there is a collusion between the law and medicine about actively choosing death. Entrenched attitudes cannot therefore change, and the choice becomes unavailable.

What can be seen, then, is that as a direct result of seeking to reach life and death decisions within a framework which is dependent on the medicalisation of the question, the law finds itself in an intellectual and ethical muddle. As Fletcher succinctly says, '[t]he courts have tried to evade the meaning of what they are doing by arguing that removing life support is not euthanasia ....Their idea is that directly causing a patient to die — by giving a fatal injection, for example — is morally wrong, but that indirectly causing the patient's death by merely ceasing to prolong life ... is not culpable because it is descriptively different.'[48] His response is to point out that '....the end or object sought is the same, and therefore the moral significance of the different means is the same'.[49]

In fact, all that differentiates the patient in PVS from the patient who seeks assistance in dying is that doctors are comfortable with the former situation and less so with the latter. By dressing the issues up in medical mystique the law does great harm to its claim to independence and justice. As Fletcher has been said, '[w]hat it comes down to is that most people, including the courts, want the end — death — in certain tragic situations, but the taboo forbids the means'.[50] Thus, alternative strategies are sought to validate the ultimate decision — strategies which, when analysed show that death is doubly medicalised. First, its timing is controlled by medicine and second it is authorised only when medicine is comfortable with the method used to achieve it. In this way, law permits 'letting die' but precludes assistance in a chosen death.

So, we are left with a situation which is ethically muddled as a result of our dependence on the doctor's perspective. The individual whose life is thought by others to lack quality may be 'allowed to die' no matter what their own views might have been. The person requiring treatment to continue his/her existence can refuse to accept it, thus ensuring death. These are both seen as permissible because the doctor is able to claim that s/he is not actively involved in the death even though there is no doubt that they play a significant role.

Doctors, however, are reluctant to play a truly active role, and for this reason (based on the Hippocratic oath) the competent person may not obtain active assistance in their choice for death. For the individual whose suffering is — as far as they are concerned — intolerable, but who is not terminally or hopelessly ill the only option is to ask for help in their death. The collusion of medicine and the law, however, leaves them with no way out. This situation is starkly illustrated by the Canadian case of Sue Rodriguez.[51]

Ms Rodriguez was a woman in her early forties suffering from amyotrophic lateral sclerosis. Her condition meant that she would ultimately (although nobody could say quite when) lose her capacity to do anything for herself; she would be totally dependent on machines to breathe and completely unable to feed or move herself. However, intellectually she would remain unimpaired — in other words, for as long as it took her to die she would be aware of the degradation and indignity to which her condition would subject her.

Ms Rodriguez wanted to stay alive for as long as she could have a quality of life which was bearable for her; she wanted more time with her children. The option of suicide could only be taken for as long as her condition had not deteriorated too far, and if taken might have denied her some precious time. She petitioned the Supreme Court to hold that the Canadian Charter of Rights and Freedoms allowed her the right to seek assistance in dying when her condition precluded suicide and had become intolerable. By a narrow majority this appeal was unsuccessful. Ms Rodriguez did eventually succeed in obtaining assistance in her death at a time of her own choosing, but only because she was able to find a doctor with the courage to act outside of the law. Who knows what additional distress was added to her suffering as a result of this; dying in the knowledge that the person who had compassionately given her the most precious gift might subsequently face prosecution.

In the United States, the issue of assisted death has also become one of great contemporary relevance. Although the State of Oregon passed legislation permitting assisted suicide in controlled circumstances,[52] the law was immediately challenged and has been held by one judge to be unconstitutional.[53] On the other hand, in a second state, a judge declared that there is a constitutional right to assisted death.[54] After these cases had been heard at state level, they reached the US Supreme Court in 1997.[55] Essentially, the Supreme Court held that a state prohibition on assisting suicide did not violate the Equal Protection Clause of the Fourteenth Amendment to the US Constitution and concluded that the debate over assisted suicide was one which properly should continue in a democratic society. Thus, the door was left open for states to enact assisted suicide laws if they so wished, and the voters of Oregon reaffirmed their commitment to their original legislation on 11 November 1997. Interestingly, the law passed this time with a much clearer majority than was obtained on the first vote. Briefly, the Northern Territory in Australia became the world's first legislature to decriminalise both assisted suicide and euthanasia before the law was overturned by the Canberra government. In The Netherlands, both euthanasia and assisted suicide continue to be tolerated in specific circumstances. In addition, in a large number of countries throughout the world, law-makers are being asked to address the current prohibition on assisting death and popular support for legal reform continues to rise.

The ambivalence of laws which allow death to be chosen only when doctors are not uncomfortable with the means used, while at the same time denying people the capacity to vindicate a competent, albeit difficult, choice beggars description. And in truth this is very much at the heart of the problem. The legal approach to passively assisted deaths shows that we do not, whatever the rhetoric, always believe that life is preferable to death. In allowing people to die by a passive route we see the sanctity of the life principle operating as it should. In other words, there is undoubtedly a value in subscribing to this principle, but it is a protection and not an obligation. The principle operates to protect those who do not wish to die; it should have no place in providing the rationale for forcing people to live when for them death is to be preferred. To allow third parties to decide that life lacks quality for someone else, for example in the case of the PVS patient, yet at the same time to deny individuals the right to make that decision for themselves, is nothing short of bizarre.

What has gone before shows an unhappy picture of a legal system seemingly in thrall to one particular approach to a subject about which people individually and collectively feel strongly. The approach of the courts is characterised by sophistry, thereby avoiding asking and answering the ultimate question — namely what are the true values and principles which society should apply to the new reality. It is, as one judge put it, attempting to fill 'the gap between old law and new medicine'.[56] Or as another commentator put it, '[t]o ease their discomforts, the courts ... take refuge in nonsensical and arbitrary statements, trying to hold on to an old way of thinking and talking while having to embrace a new way to meet new realities.'[57]

And new realities there are. Although of little more than anecdotal value, there is no doubt that the attitudes of many people towards their own inevitable death have changed. A life without quality may be the outcome of heroic medical intervention, but many would prefer not to live it. For example, a Harris Poll[58] in 1995 showed that in a survey of 1,250 Americans, of the 94 per cent who had heard of Dr Kevorkian (who admits to have helped many patients to die and who has been the subject of extensive media coverage) 58 per cent approved of what he was doing. Existence in a state of permanent insentience is possible, but many would avoid it at all costs. The same Harris Poll showed that doctors by a margin of 70 per cent to 27 per cent believed that the law should allow them to assist in the death of a dying patient who was in severe distress. Even the medical perception is changing, with 54 per cent of a recent survey of doctors and pharmacists in the United Kingdom also favouring a change in the law to permit assisted suicide in certain circumstances.[59]

It is certainly the case that it is medicine which forces us to address these issues, but this does not make them medical matters, nor does it suggest that the historical constraints of medical ethics are the best or the only standpoint from which to proceed. But, for as long as laws and judges find the medical model to be a convenient way of proclaiming one thing in principle and practising another, general societal values are ignored or distorted. It is not the purpose of medicine that is at stake, but rather a higher one. As an eminent Australian judge has said, '[t]o insist upon the prolongation of life, as nothing more than the coursing of blood and bodily functions, and to do so in circumstances of intractable and irremedial pain, is so offensive to the very purpose of human life that it calls out for relief'.[60] Equally, to determine whether or not life shall not be prolonged on the basis of what is comfortable within the medical model is to subvert ethical values to the prejudices of the clinical.

Although some jurisdictions have moved further away from the purely medical model than others, medicine has a strong and crucial input in virtually every decision reached by courts. Even in those countries which tolerate or have legalised assisted suicide or euthanasia, the role of the doctor is pivotal. Although we would undoubtedly wish to see an input from those who can with varying degrees of certainty tell us what quality of life we may expect and what care is available to us, many, if not most, people would regard this as informative rather than definitive of the issue.

Equally, we have a right to expect internal consistency from our laws — a consistency which is threatened when decisions are based on flawed preconceptions or inappropriate rationales. Yet, it would be no solution to return to the days when these issues were out of the public eye. Even although decisions about the end of one's life may ideally be made in privacy or with the comfort of the involvement of loved ones and the professionals who care for us, the law still has a role to play in respecting the values of the individual and the interests of society. Few countries in the West realistically hold on to an absolute prohibition on decisions at the end of life. The growing recognition of the value of advance directives, the admission that euthanasia is practised even where it is illegal and the efforts by some to have their choice for death legally endorsed, demonstrate that societies have moved on.

The taboos surrounding death now are more frequently confronted and challenged and the impetus for personal control of death is a logical extension of the drive to control life. If the law is to play its part in realising human aspirations it must rid itself of the old-fashioned and increasingly criticised dependence on medicine and confront the new reality head on. In the view of many, this can only be done by legislative intervention. Not only can this option be seen as reflecting the democratic will, it can also serve to disengage law from its venerable ally, medicine, and focus the state's capacity to control and regulate human behaviour firmly where it should be — on the interests of its citizens.

8 Controlling or Conceding the Future?

The capacities of modern medicine are nothing short of awe inspiring. The preceding chapters have shown the extent to which, from cradle to grave, even pre-cradle to post-grave, what doctors know and what they can do will intimately affect us. Linked in a close embrace, we are 'participants in a cultural process, a fundamental *mentality,* overvaluing the contributions of medical science and technology to the pursuit of human happiness and well-being, and believing medicine's promises to eliminate human suffering and mortality'.[1] Moreover, we are all deeply affected by the kinds of questions which science and medicine ask. For example, it is doubtless the case that many people feel that circumventing infertility is on balance a good thing, but had medicine never questioned the possibility, we would not now be struggling with the dilemmas which have inevitably emerged. Similarly, if technology had not developed to the extent that life can be sustained in those who would otherwise have died, the harrowing problems concerning when treatment should be discontinued would not be taxing our morality and our consciences.

Of course, medicine and science must ask questions and the fact that moral dilemmas arise as a result of them is no reason for preferring stasis. Antibiotics, anaesthesia and a whole host of major steps forward would never have been developed if doctors and scientists had not been enquiring, and the world would have been significantly poorer. Indeed, doctors are arguably obliged to test the frontiers of their capacities by undertaking research which will inform and enhance both current and future health care. This is a professional obligation as well as a legitimate public expectation.

What has been suggested, however, is that we should beware a too simplistic assumption that advance is value-free — that it can be attained without cost. As Callahan says, 'The most potent social impact of medical advancement is the way it reshapes our notions of what it is to have a life .... The greatest attraction of technological innovation is its promise of first breaking the barriers of natural, biological constraints, and then moving on to a dismantling of the cultural attitudes and institutions designed to live within these barriers.'[2] Given the enormity of this proposition, it may be that in some cases mature reflection suggests that the cost is too high or that the society in which we live is under-equipped to manage the consequences. I am no scientific luddite, but the examples which I have already discussed suggest that more often than not the latter is true. In part, this reflects the distance between the layperson and the professional, but it also reflects the lack of public involvement in matters which shape our world, and in particular it mandates a form of legal involvement hitherto undreamed of.

What has been suggested is that to date the law's response to incredibly complex developments and decisions has been ambivalent. The decision whether or not legal intervention is appropriate and whether it comes in the best possible form has been reached by *ad hocery* rather than on the basis of mature reflection. Moreover, those operating the legal system, perhaps themselves overwhelmed by the subtleties and complexities of the issues raised, have often opted out of addressing the fundamental human rights issues by medicalising the question. Having done so, they are then apparently satisfied with handing over decision-making responsibility to those with the clinical or scientific expertise, but whose capacity to reach ethical conclusions is at best no better than that of anyone else and whose professional enthusiasm and ambitions may serve to colour their judgements.

Nor will these dilemmas simply disappear with experience. Assisted reproductive technologies continue to advance, with moral decisions being made, and issues of human rights raised, by pre-conception counselling and pre-implantation diagnosis. End of life decisions are regularly taken, permitting one group of citizens the power of life and death over another, within a legal framework whose approach is most kindly categorised as pragmatic. Yet all of these things matter to us, as individuals as well as communities. The extent to which people would, if they were aware of it, genuinely be satisfied that the collusion of powerful medicine and acquiescent law in fact predicts and controls many of our most basic rights, is a matter for speculation.

But some anecdotal evidence is available which suggests that, when asked, people would prefer to have more control over their lives rather than less. Opinion polls from many countries, for example, uniformly show a majority of people in favour of legalising euthanasia or assisted suicide.[3] In some countries this has been translated into legislation, albeit only in a very few. However, what these polls demonstrate is that — if the question is asked — there emerges a sense that our lives are ours and that we should have the greater say in what happens to them. People's involvement in shaping medical advances or deciding when to stop is, however, rare — the questions are seldom, if ever, asked.

But it is not only in addressing what questions should be asked that the public is disenfranchised. Once something is available it is in demand. Thus, it seems almost blasphemous to suggest that a moratorium might be a viable way of obtaining the opinions of those whom it will affect. The craving for advance may sometimes make those who ask for caution seem out of step, irrelevant or downright malicious. There will always be one group for whom the advance seems to hold out hope and to suggest that others should be involved in its control or in limiting its availability may be viewed as heartless.

We are, unfortunately, often ill-informed and therefore our voices often weak. Unsurprisingly, of course, some of the ethical dilemmas which emerge as technology advances could probably not have been predicted at the inception of the technology, although I would argue that many of them could have been. There is an underlying set of values and interests which have been shown to emerge whatever the topic being considered in this book. New developments will be likely to share some of these at least, even if more emerge as time goes on, and these could be used to provide the basis for the inception of an informed debate.

It has never been more important that this lesson is learned, because medicine's new frontiers are already upon us. Science's pioneers are already tackling challenges and posing questions which — even 20 years ago — would have been unthinkable, questions which for many belong in the world of science fiction and not science fact. But we should already have learned that yesterday's story is today's reality in this rapidly expanding world. Fiction writers have made millions from stories of perfect societies made up of cloned 'designer' people. They have titillated our imaginations with warnings of genetic underclasses, with the creation of uncontrollable monsters from small DNA samples, of scientists in white coats plotting to overthrow the world by releasing genetically modified organisms.

Fantasies they may be, but possible they certainly are. Perhaps the biggest, and certainly one of the most ambitious scientific projects of all time is now rendering such things part of a potential reality. What will prevent their translation into the real world is the extent to which they are controlled. Given what has been discussed in previous chapters, the question must be soberly asked — how confident are we in the mechanisms available to control? How sure are we that the current research is asking questions, the answers to which we want to know? How comfortable are we that when all that can be known is known we will have either relevant or sufficiently sophisticated mechanisms in place to minimise the possibility of abuse?

The challenge is of course posed by the Human Genome Project (HGP)[4] and the so-called 'new genetics'. The 'new' genetics will translate the information gleaned from the Genome Project into reality — hopefully by the provision of therapy. The use of the word 'new' is designed to distance current science from the history of abuse of elementary genetic knowledge and certainly it seems unthinkable that the excesses of the early part of this century would be repeated. However, even given this, it would be naïve in the extreme to believe that there are, and will be, no profound moral dilemmas raised both by the acquisition and by the use of genetic information. In this respect, genetic knowledge provides the clearest reason yet for serious evaluation of the argument which has run throughout this book.

The purpose of the Human Genome Project has been said to be '[a]cquiring complete knowledge of the organization, structure and function of the human genome — the master blueprint of each of us ...'[5] The acquisition of this knowledge will tell us more about ourselves than we have ever known. Unless properly controlled, it will open up a Pandora's box resulting in consequences as yet unthought of or unthinkable. Of course, it is information which also gives immense benefits. As Robinson has said:

This 15-year project, costing $3 to $5 billion, [US dollars] will involve researchers around the world. Achieving its aim

— to locate and discover the sequence of the genes that make up the human genome — will prepare the way for matching genes with gene products and for learning what these products do and how genes are regulated.[6]

In other words, some outcomes of the knowledge gained will be to explain disease processes, to find ways of modifying genetic structures and hopefully matching this understanding with products which will make therapy or cure available. The benefits may, therefore, be immeasurable, since the toll of suffering caused directly or indirectly by genetic disorders cannot be underestimated. The British Medical Association (BMA), for example, have estimated that 'Genetic and pre-genetic diseases affect one in every twenty people by the age of 25 and perhaps as many as two in three people during their lifetime'.[7]

Not every disorder will necessarily have dire consequences, but manifestly if this estimate is accurate, many people will suffer some problems which advances in genetic knowledge may help to alleviate. But two issues require preliminary comment. The first is the use of the word 'disorder'. Commonly, aberrant genes are described as 'defective', and the notion of defect is one which conjures up undesirability. The language used, therefore, is of considerable importance, since one outcome of undesirability might be elimination. The second matter relates to the faith that by discovering something we will be able to treat it. It is accepted that although '[u]nderstanding does not always presage more effective treatment ... the promise is high'.[8] Equally, however, it cannot be assumed that knowledge will lead inevitably to cure, and at present the therapeutic shortfall is quite significant.

As has been shown in earlier chapters, we must beware the trap of assuming that either the search for knowledge or the knowledge itself is in some way value free. Scientific enquiry may be shaped by a number of factors ranging from the fortuitous to the financial. In respect of genetic knowledge, the race to come first will provide significant advantages for those who achieve it. As Galloway says, 'Whoever gets the human genome data first will decide what will happen to them, and will be in an unassailable position to dictate terms over its commercial, including its medical, exploitation'.[9] Given the importance of genetic information, the power of control is a strong encouragement for individuals and countries to be and stay ahead of the race.

But those who are searching for that knowledge, no matter how benign or disinterested their intentions, will also have to face the fact that its acquisition will be a 'source of intriguing, and at times formidable, ethical issues.'[10] And, despite the view of the BMA that 'biotechnology and genetic information are in themselves morally neutral',[11] I would suggest that, while the uses to which that information are put may be the more problematic situation, the mere holding of the information is in itself of great ethical concern.

Seldom is information free from moral interpretation — the very fact that it is sought suggests that it is worth having, and if it is worth having then in itself it has power. In any event, even if merely neutrally recorded, the mere fact of its storage renders it usable. Thus, it is not possible to separate out the gaining of knowledge from its use, although the latter may seem to be more susceptible of control. As The Royal College of Physicians of London said: 'The problems of gathering genetic information seem to fall into two main areas. The first of these concerns the problem of whether a particular investigation should be undertaken at all. The second concerns the obstacles that may be encountered once a decision to investigate has been made.'[12]

That there are many ethical dilemmas is not in doubt, and some will be considered below, but there is one further issue in respect of genetic information which must be dealt with briefly. The HGP was initially designed as a government sponsored, international collaborative venture. From the beginning it was recognised that problems might arise, and in the United States a percentage of funding was set aside to address the ethical, social and legal consequences of the research outcome. Equally, however, we have occasionally seen internecine scientific squabbling, and a dramatic rush to patent rather than share discoveries, potentially 'undermining many of the traditional and desirable aspects of scientific work and collaboration'.[13] In addition, private funding is increasingly becoming involved in the research. The problems of this were pointed to by Schmidtke with some prescience. As he said:

> if the government permits, and even provokes by lack of funding, a situation where basic research, including genetic research, is undertaken in commercially oriented laboratories, this can result in knowledge of the human genome being owned partially, and at least temporarily, by private individuals. Such circumstances are potentially dangerous because knowledge is closely associated with power and because ... knowledge and the power associated with it are uncontrollable.[14]

Of course, there are many good things which will come out of the Human Genome Project and scaremongering is an inappropriate response to the 'new' genetics. So too, however, is complacency. As Engelhardt points out:

> We must be aware of the possible uses and misuses that may be made of biotechnology in the future ... but it distorts our thinking about the moral or human implications of genetic therapy and other forms of biotechnology if we always

discuss them in terms of extreme and unreal possibilities. These exaggerated scenarios make imaginative science fiction and sensational journalism and exciting polemic, but they do not help to advance the truth.[15]

Maddox would go even further, claiming that 'the widespread fear of genetics cannot be justified. On the contrary, the research community should speak out strongly to defend the good sense of what it is about.'[16] Whichever position is adopted, from the moderate to the extreme, one thing is obvious. Genetic knowledge will affect us all, in ways which may not at first sight be entirely obvious and the use to which it will be put will result in individuals being 'genetically laid bare and vulnerable as never before.'[17]

Of course, if benefits outweigh costs then our calculation as to what risks we are ready assume may shift. The potential hazards of genetic information might pale into insignificance if we knew that the consequences of having it would be both controlled and therapeutic. Again, therefore, a vital question mark hangs over the role played by society in managing the information and its sequelae, a point which will be returned to later. For the moment, though, it is worth concentrating on the question of therapy. It has already been suggested that there is a therapeutic shortfall — a difference between what we know and what we can do about it. Doubtless, over time this gap may narrow, but we cannot be sure precisely what impact genetics will have on health. As the BMA has said:

At this relatively early stage in the development of applied genetics it is too early to be certain precisely how extensive its benefits may become. While great prospective benefits for medical science have been claimed by some protagonists, others have argued that genetic modification may have a great deal to offer to medical science but may be of less practical value to patient care.[18]

Would this thought, if borne out, modify the enthusiasm with which we might otherwise greet genetic developments? One further issue is of importance. At the moment scientists are still finding things out, but the drive is also on to find the therapy which will eradicate the conditions which are genetically determined. Some would see this drive as being naïve, in that genetic modifications do not invariably presage illness — we all carry some harmful genes and yet may live a full life, terminated by factors which have nothing to do with our genetic make-up. Yet, for some members of the community, the knowledge that we carry the gene for breast cancer or Huntington's Disease will doubtless lead to a demand for increased research. This is entirely understandable, but it also means that human beings will — until therapies are established — be increasingly the subjects of research and experimentation, a subject already fraught with difficulties.

Some of the research will be carried out on adult, competent citizens and this is generally regarded as acceptable so long as they are fully informed about the risks and benefits associated with their involvement. But in all research, whether or not it is genetic, there is a lingering doubt about the extent to which anyone makes a truly free choice to become a research subject when their own health is at risk. Be that as it may, we have absorbed this into our ethical framework and seem reasonably comfortable with it. However, some conditions will involve screening and testing of the unborn or young children. Consent in their cases is infinitely more problematic — indeed, it is unobtainable. Yet, because of the nature of genes, which are shared with the entire family, screening of the very young may help the rest of the family and also future patients.

The question must be asked whether or not this too can be readily encapsulated within an ethical framework. This may in part also depend on the outcome — in other words the justification will be consequentialist rather than rights-based. But doubts remain. As Davis said:

> we cannot assume that making use of present patients for the good of future patients is ethically legitimate, particularly since the patients concerned are in no position to volunteer .... It could be said of molecular biology that, insofar as human genetics is concerned, it has gained a scientific empire but not yet found its real clinical role.[19]

The potential areas of concern are too wide and too diverse to be considered in depth, but some of them merit consideration before a conclusion can be reached about the appropriate response. Some have already been touched upon in other chapters. For example, the reproductive revolution, which has devised methods of circumventing infertility, has also led to increased capacities to screen and test the human embryo or foetus for genetic disorders. It is admitted that the logical outcome, in the absence of available therapy, of such procedures is that the embryo or foetus concerned will not be permitted to mature.

Without entering into the abortion debate again, it is clear that the very provision of testing with termination as the outcome will simply be unacceptable to some people. But even those who tolerate abortion may feel some unease about its expanded use, and in particular about the mind set which underlies termination based on disability or disorder. Naturally, most people wish to have a healthy child, but the likely increased wastage of embryos and foetuses which will result from the application of genetic knowledge may nonetheless be of concern. It has been reported, for example, that women in the United States have been terminating pregnancies in which doctors have found chromosomal abnormalities, even although there is no evidence that they would result in a disabled or disabled child.[20] Pressure may be put on women to terminate pregnancies which are affected in some way, and what has been called 'intergenerational justice' may seem to mandate that women (and their partners) should refrain from reproducing if they carry deleterious genes.

Pre-implantation diagnosis is now also available, although in the UK, 'By 1995, fewer than 150 cases of pre-implantation diagnosis had been undertaken'.[21] Given the availability of skills and resources, and in the light of advances in genetic knowledge, it seems likely that this number will increase. Again, the desire to have a healthy child cannot be minimised, but there are subtleties about pre-implantation diagnosis which, even for the most ardent supporter of choice in reproduction, throw up moral questions which must be addressed.

One of the benefits of diagnosing conditions before the embryo is implanted is that — at this stage — for many people the embryo has no moral status or at least a very reduced one. It is not the attribution of status in se that is significant, though, because many people (and indeed the law itself) would not attribute status to the embryo or foetus no matter the stage of its development. Rather it is that the judgements made about the pre-implanted embryo, taking account of its reduced status, may serve to enhance discrimination. If we are unconcerned about the embryo before implantation, then we may choose to screen for, and then screen out, a whole range of conditions which might — were the embryo already implanted — be regarded as inappropriate to look for or insufficiently serious to merit a pregnancy termination, thus reinforcing discrimination against others who suffer from the same condition.

Moreover, the mere fact of carrying a gene which predisposes to a particular condition neither inevitably predicts its onset nor tells us when the onset will be. Thus, if the gene is for a late-onset condition in particular, too easy discarding of the embryo may deny that embryo the potential of many years of happy and productive life, solely on the basis of its 'defect'. The uncertainties of genetic prediction therefore pose additional dilemmas for this debate.

Pre-natal screening is, of course, more readily available — indeed, in many countries it is encouraged. But Hubbard and Wald, for example, suggest that 'Most prenatal tests offer little precise information. They can suggest problems, but cannot say how significant these problems may be.'[22] Moreover, in similar vein to the comments concerning pre-implantation diagnosis, they caution that 'Genetic predictions, like all medical tests, involve setting arbitrary norms. People, or foetuses, who fall outside them as by definition "abnormal", irrespective of whether they exhibit noticeable symptoms or whether these symptoms are particularly debilitating.'[23] The lessons to be learned from this caution are clear.

Moreover, genetic knowledge may affect the very reproductive decision itself, either by scaring people out of reproduction or by categorising them as unfit for parenting. The historical use of this latter concept has already been described, but it has manifested itself even more recently. Skene, for example, notes that 'In a pilot genetic screening project in Greece, carriers of the gene that causes sickle cell disease were stigmatised by their community and considered ineligible for marriage, except to other carriers'.[24] That such discrimination is in part based on ignorance does not mean that it will not commend itself to some individuals and to some communities. As Charlesworth said, 'Feminist critics of the new reproductive technologies have shown how difficult it is to divorce these technologies from their ideological contexts, and the same is true of genetics and genetic technologies'.[25]

It is not only at the beginning of life that genetics may have an impact. For those who know their genetic inheritance there may also be an awareness of the way in which they will die, and a corresponding increase in demand for choice at the end of life. However, with few exceptions, the law in most countries will not endorse the competent request of an individual for assistance in dying, no matter the evidence from opinion polls that a majority would wish to see the law changed. Even although sentencing in 'mercy killing' cases tends to be lenient, those who are aware of the dreadfulness of their impending death may well be in the vanguard of a new movement to wrest control of one's own dying into one's own power. To this extent, genetic knowledge would add to the sum of values encapsulated within the concept of autonomy, assuming that pressure for legal change was successful.

However, if laws do not change, there is a second danger, namely that people will be kept alive in circumstances where they would prefer death. As Davis has said,

> Along with the triumphs of modern advances in medicine a tragic side-product has been the use of heroic measures to keep alive bodies that are only a source of prolonged misery for the individuals and their families .... If some of the applications of gene therapy should provide prolongation of life without restoration of reasonable quality, one would hope that such cases will not automatically become subjects for this most extreme of heroic therapies.[26]

Discrimination is, clearly, one of the major possible downsides of the genetic revolution, and it can occur outside of areas which are traditionally seen as medical. When information is knowable, then it is tempting to demand that it is known. For the individual who may prefer not to know his or her genetic inheritance, pressures may nonetheless be brought to bear in the interests of others or of the state to find out that information.

Insurance agencies and employers for example may seek information for a variety of reasons. They may wish to make sound actuarial calculations of risk for the purpose of insurance premium-setting or they may wish to ensure that the employee is safe in any given workplace. However, there may also be a more sinister side to this quest for information. Insurers may decline to take the risk and create an uninsurable underclass. In contemporary society, the inability to obtain insurance for life or health purposes can mean the difference between a life with quality and a life with little or none. In countries whose health care system is largely insurance-based, it may mean — as it already does — that increasing numbers of people fall outside of any safety net; that the elderly will not be treated; that ante-natal care will not be undertaken; that people will die for the lack of elementary care.

The inability to obtain insurance may, therefore, be a more directly life-threatening event than would be the genetic disorder itself. Some countries have attempted to tackle this problem. In The Netherlands, for example, a moratorium was declared by which the insurance industry agreed not to ask for genetic information about people whose policies were for an amount below a certain figure.[27] In the US, the Insurance Task Force recommended that genetic information should not be sought,[28] and in the UK the House of Commons Select Committee on Science and Technology gave the insurance industry one year (now spent) to come up with an acceptable policy or face legislation.[29] Although the industry in the UK failed to meet this deadline, an expert geneticist has now been employed to raise the quality of decision-making and the interpretation of genetic information — and a committee has been established to address the industry's decisions from an ethical perspective.

Employers too may have an interest in obtaining access to information about the genetic make-up of their employees. In the UK, for example, at the moment, there is no law which would preclude employers from seeking such information, although some may feel that it would be a good idea to have one. Of course, genetic information could be useful in protecting the health of an employee, but it could also be valuable to the employer in reaching employment decisions themselves. Those deemed to be genetically defective might be denied employment opportunities if this information comes to the attention of a prospective employer, or promotion opportunities if already in employment.

The Nuffield Council on Bioethics feels strongly about this. In their view, 'people should be excluded from employment opportunities only where this is shown to be absolutely necessary. We see no reason why people should be required to undergo genetic screening unless the illness or condition will present a serious danger to third parties.'[30] Nonetheless, there are undoubtedly arguments which have been, and will be, put forward which would lend support to workplace screening programmes, yet Murray suggests that 'The early proponents of workplace genetic screening did not foresee the political, economic, and ethical complexities'[31] which such screening would raise.

But the fact that arguments **can** be made by insurers and employers, and doubtless others, that the genetic inheritance of an individual is information which is of value to them and to which they are therefore entitled, disguises the dangers lurking underneath their ready acceptance. If the information is valuable, then it is valuable *in se*. If it is necessary to the making of sound actuarial calculations or to appropriate employment decisions, then it is all too easy to slide from a position which says it is desirable to know into one which says it is essential to know. Although not yet seriously proposed, compulsion hovers on the horizon. And compulsion is an integral part of the argument. If the insurance industry will collapse without access to this information, and if this is a bad thing, then why should we allow individuals not to know the information which is relevant to its survival, or if they know it why should we not be allowed to demand that it is disclosed?

The right of the individual to privacy is seriously threatened if this logic is followed. Equally, any right not to know is washed away. The traditions of privacy and confidentiality in health care are themselves threatened by the advances currently being made by geneticists, precisely because there is, as yet, no serious effort being made by the law to underscore the values which inform civilised societies. Certainly, balancing of interests may be needed but balance cannot be achieved without knowing the weights on either side of the scale.

There are, of course, many other examples which could be used to show the potential of genetic information as a vehicle for discrimination and displacement of the individual. This does not detract from the genuine benefits which we can reasonably expect to reap from the genetic revolution, but it does urge caution and demands thorough analysis. The BMA notes that for some genetics is 'incorrigibly reductionist',[32] reducing what it is to be a human being to a set of cells. But as Charlesworth cautions, 'A theory of human nature should also provide some account of the relationship between the "given" biological and physical constraints on human life and the creative element which enables us to elaborate and transform biological dispositions and tendencies and inclinations and give them distinctly human meanings.'[33] Or as Rose et al. put it, 'Humanity cannot be cut adrift from its own biology, but neither is it enchained by it.'[34]

This is a particularly important point and one which endorses the approach taken in this book. The temptation to reduce humanity to a collection of cells disvalues what is special and unique about the individual. It poses a danger to people's inner sense of worth, to their sense of personal responsibility. It disenfranchises people by rendering them powerless rather than powerful — victims rather than moral agents. Moreover, it encourages the dominance of a way of thinking and a set of values which undoubtedly have importance but which call for fundamentally different forms of enquiry from the moral or the philosophical, and which must therefore be kept firmly in their place.

To be sure, it may well be that the potential fears about genetics are a direct result of societal ignorance about its meaning and content. Pleas for the education of the public are commonplace in this area, for a number of reasons, not least that genetic information is not as set in stone as some would have us believe. Understanding that 'genetic conditions involve a largely unpredictable interplay of many factors and processes'[35] may serve to ensure that simplistic assumptions are avoided.

But to understand even this apparently elementary point, it may be that some scientific knowledge is required, and this the public by and large lacks. Indeed, the subject is so complex that even other scientists may find it difficult to absorb. Yet understanding is empowerment — not understanding of the intricacies of molecular biology necessarily, but rather understanding based on the legitimate demand that science and scientists divest themselves of jargon and explain the human consequences of what they are asking and what they are doing. If we are to reap the rich harvest of genetics without being swamped by its potential for harm, we must be involved in its progress, alert to its goals and become the designers and monitors of its values.

Genetics possibly highlights in the starkest possible way the hidden dangers of permitting ourselves to rest snug in the certainty that 'they' are doing the right thing — 'they' are also 'us', and what 'they' do will have substantial, often intimate, consequences for each individual and the community of which they are a part. Genetics can pose the tensions between science and the individual in 3D — despair, disempowerment and discrimination. Properly handled, it can expand capacities, enhance well-being and permit growth. The real power of science and medicine lies not in what **they** know but in what **we** don't know. The real threat to human values and human rights lies in the transfer of authority to any given discipline.

It may well be, as some would suggest, that reaction is better than anticipation. The BMA, for example say that although 'At first sight anticipation of risks seems far superior to the trial and error of reactive regulation …. Very often our understanding of hazards is most readily advanced by analysis of actual events, sometimes involving accidents.'[36] And Davis has argued that, 'In a world in which science and technology are changing our patterns of living and our problems with unprecedented speed, resilience in response … is likely to be more effective than efforts at detailed anticipation.'[37]

These are seductive arguments, but they miss the point. First, they presume that stopping progress is not an option, yet from what has been said here it must surely be considered to be every bit as feasible as blindly following the path mapped out for us by modern medicine and science. Second, they merge the technical into the ethical. It is not to the details of technology that this book has addressed itself. Rather it is to the underpinning values that we must look. These values are unaffected by advances in any discipline, because they underlie what it is to be a member of a society; they respect what it is to be free, uncoerced and involved in our world, and they invite participation from everyone.

Most particularly, however, by categorising dilemmas as medical, society as a whole, and the law in particular, has shuffled off responsibility and has endangered human rights. No matter one's dissatisfaction with the law, it remains true that

> Society will expect the law to protect its wider ideals and, in particular, the individual citizen, from the excesses of over-enthusiastic doctors and scientists, greedy corporations and immoral profiteers and manipulators. The law will have to balance the need for future research against the need to protect society from its dangers and evils.[38]

However, this the law cannot do until it disentangles human issues from medical ones. It is not the mechanics of the law's response which are so important as its content — a content informed by concern for liberty, for the protection of the vulnerable and for the reinforcement of ideals. Schmidtke has said that 'Scientists are at least no better and no worse than the society of which they are members, and criticism of science is part of legitimate social critique'.[39] This book is intended to contribute to that critique by describing the complex and interrelated dilemmas which modern medicine poses. It is designed to alert the reader to the potential for the inappropriate use of decision-making models which are inimical to the protection of human values and human rights. For better or for worse, it is to the law in all its forms that we look for assurance that these values do predominate, and we may well feel on reflection that in this the law has to date failed. The collusion of the professions has minimised their capacity to respect and safeguard those whose lives they affect, sometimes invade. Their fundamental ethics are open to challenge as never before. In a hard-hitting critique of professional ethics, Koehn sums up the position as she sees it: 'I cannot think it mere coincidence that prostitution has become known as "the most ancient profession" at the turn of this century, the era in which professions exhibit every sign of becoming "the most recent prostitution"'.[40]

Unless a coherent and intelligent reassessment is made of the dangers of medicalisation, we will become less free, less independent and less proactive, infantilised by a comfortable alliance of two of the most powerful institutions in the state — medicine and the law. The effect of the medicalisation of the human condition is manifest, affecting every step taken after the medical model is engaged. As Miller says, 'Once a person has undergone the medical "rite of passage" he has ceased to be an agent and has become a patient — someone who suffers not only his disease but the various procedures by which it is cured.'[41] No less than an intellectual revolution is needed to prevent this from happening. The sophistication of current medical advances, and the speed with which they are taking place, mandate that revolution sooner rather than later.

Notes

Preface

1 *Times Law Report*, 8 May 1998

1 Setting the Scene

1. Crichton, M., *Jurassic Park*, London, Century, 1991, p.312
2. Cm 249/1987
3. para 1.2, p.1
4. Schwartz, R.L., 'Life Style, Health Status, and Distributive Justice', in Grubb, A. and Mehlman, J. (eds), *Justice and Health Care: Comparative Perspectives*, Chichester, John Wiley & Sons, 1995, at p.225.
5. loc.cit., at pp.225–6
6. Illich, I., *Limits to Medicine. Medical Nemesis: The Expropriation of Health*, Harmondsworth, Penguin, 1977, p.11
7. Illich, *Limits to Medicine*, 1977, at p.123
8. By including social and other forms of well-being into the definition of health, WHO has been criticised both for the breadth and therefore vagueness of the definition and for potentially medicalising personal, social and political phenomena.
9. Kennedy, I., *Treat Me Right: Essays in Medical Law and Ethics*, Oxford, Clarendon Press, 1988 (reprinted 1994), at p.23
10. Anleu, S.R., 'Reproductive Autonomy: Infertility, Deviance and Conceptive Technology', in Petersen, K. (ed.), *Law and Medicine* (Special Issue of *Law in Context*) Vol. 11(2), 1993, La Trobe University Press, 1994, 17, at p.19
11. loc.cit., at p.21
12. op.cit. at p.51

13. Katz, J., *The Silent World of Doctor and Patient*, New York, The Free Press, 1984, at p.46.

14. Mechanic, D., 'The Comparative Study of Health Care Delivery Systems', *Annual Review of Sociology* 1:43 (1975), at p.55

15. op.cit., at pp.13–14

16. Turner, B.S., *Medical Power and Social Knowledge*, London, Sage Publications, 1987, at p.154

17. at p.155

18. id.

19. op.cit., at p.174

20. Pellegrino, E.D., 'Intersections of Western Biomedical Ethics and World Culture: Problematic and Possibility', *Cambridge Quarterly of Healthcare Ethics* (1992) 3 191, at pp.191–2

21. Pellegrino, loc.cit., at p.192

22. Kass, L.R., *Toward a More Natural Science: Biology and Human Affairs*, New York, The Free Press, 1985, at p.25

23. Pellegrino, E.D. and Thomasma, D.C., *A Philosophical Basis of Medical Practice*, New York, OPU, 1981, at pp.viii-ix

24. See, for example, Hart, H.L.A., *Law, Liberty and Morality*, Oxford, OUP, 1963, particularly at p.79. 'The central mistake is a failure to distinguish the acceptable principle that political power is best entrusted to the majority from the unacceptable claim that what the majority do with that power is beyond criticism and must never be resisted. No one can be a democrat who does not accept the first of these, but no democrat need accept the second.'

25. Franklin, U., 'New Threats to Human Rights Through Science and Technology — The Need for Standards', in Mahoney, K.E. and Mahoney, P. (eds), *Human Rights in the Twenty-first Century*, Dordrecht, Kluwer Academic Publishers, 1993, 733, at p.733

26. Katz, op.cit., at p.28

27. op.cit., at p.20

28. loc.cit., at p.734

29. McVeigh, S. and Wheeler, S. 'Introduction', in McVeigh, S. and Wheeler, S. (eds), *Health and Medical Regulation*, Aldershot, Dartmouth, 1992, at p.vi

30. id.

31. HL Paper 21–1, London, HMSO, 1994

32. para 272, p.56

33. id.

34. In the UK this is done by use of the 'Bolam Test' derived from the case of *Bolam* v. *Friern Hospital Management Committee* [1957] 2 All ER 118, which broadly says that if a doctor acts in accordance with a practice accepted as reasonable by responsible body of medical opinion, then he or she will not be negligent. The law, therefore, sets the standard, but the content is arguably set by doctors themselves. Broadly similar rules apply in the majority of US states although some have followed the rule derived from the case of *Canterbury* v. *Spence* 464 F 2d 772 (1972) which is more patient-centred. A recent Australian judgement in the case of *Rogers* v. *Whitaker* (1992) 109 ALR 625 saw what may be the beginning of a move away from the professionally based test in that country. For a discussion of the problems of applying the Bolam Test, see McLean, S.A.M., *A Patient's Right to Know: Information Disclosure, The Doctor and The Law*, Aldershot, Dartmouth, 1989

35. Pellegrino and Thomasma, op.cit., at pp.viii-ix

36. Kass, op.cit., at p.43

37. McLean, S.A.M., 'Law Versus Morality', in Szawarski, Z. and Evans, D. (eds), *Solidarity, Justice and Health Care Priorities*, Linkoping, LCC, Linkoping University, 1993, 110, at p.119

38. Furrow, B.R., 'Forcing Rescue: the Landscape of Health Care Provider Obligations to Treat Patients', in Grubb and Mehlman, op.cit.,41, at p.43

39. Morgan, D. and Neilsen, L., 'Dangerous Liaisons? Law, Technology, Reproduction and European Ethics', in McVeigh and Wheeler, op.cit., 52, at p.55

40. Katz, op.cit., at p.59

41. McLean, loc.cit., at p.112

2 The Reproduction Revolution — Liberation or Liability?

1. For discussion, see McLean, S.A.M., 'The Right to Reproduce', in Campbell, et al. (eds), *Human Rights: From Rhetoric to Reality*, Oxford, Basil Blackwell, 1986.

2. c.f. *Skinner* v. *Oklahoma* 316 US 636 (1942); *Griswold* v. *Connecticut* 381

US 479 (1965)

3. Mason, J.K., *Medico-Legal Aspects of Reproduction and Parenthood*, Aldershot, Dartmouth, 1990, at p.187

4. Most commonly the provision of services to the unmarried; see for example, the Human Fertilisation and Embryology Act 1990 (UK) s.13(5). The provision of services to those who are unmarried or who have not been in a stable heterosexual relationship for five years is outlawed in Western Australia

5. Edwards, R. and Sharpe, D., 'Social Values and Research in Human Embryology', *Nature*, 231, 87 (1971), at p.87

6. For further discussion, see Morgan, D. and Lee, R.G., *Blackstone's Guide to the Human Fertilisation and Embryology Act 1990*, London, Blackstone Press, 1991

7. Woollett, A., 'Psychological Aspects of Infertility and Infertility Investigations', in Nicolson, R. and Ussher, J. (eds), *The Psychology of Women's Health and Health Care*, The Macmillan Press, 1992, 152, at p.165

8 Ussher, J., 'Reproductive Rhetoric and the Blaming of the Body', in Nicolson and Ussher, op.cit., 31, at pp.47–8

9. Plato, *Timaeus*, quoted by Veith, *Hysteria: The History of a Disease*, University of Chicago Press, 1964, at p.7

10. c.f. Rowland, R., *Living Laboratories: Women and Reproductive Technology*, London, Cedar, 1992. At p.5 she sets the scene: 'A history can be traced of the continuing battle between the two social groups, men and women, over the control of women's fertility and procreative potential. This battle is drawn around race and class lines, and governments constantly develop systems structured to control which women have children, when, how and how many. The new reproductive technologies extend their power to do so in ways unimaginable a few decades ago.'

11. Engelhardt, H.T., *The Foundations of Bioethics*, Oxford, OUP, 1986, at p.241

12. Gorovitz, S., *Doctors' Dilemmas: Moral Conflict and Medical Care*, New York, OUP, 1982, at p.168

13. Beecher, H., 'Ethics and Clinical Research', *New England J. of Medicine*, Vol.274 part 24, 1966, 1354

14. c.f. McLean, *loc.cit.*

15. Murray, T.H., 'Ethical Issues in Human Genome Research', *The FASEB Journal*, Vol. 5, January 1991, 55, at p.59.

16. For further discussion, see Gordon, L., *Woman's Body, Woman's Right*, Harmondsworth, Penguin, 1977.

17. Meyers, D., *The Human Body and the Law*, Edinburgh, Edinburgh University Press, 1971, at p.29

18. *Buck v. Bell* 274 US 200 (1927)

19. at p.207

20. Sherwin, S., *No Longer Patient: Feminist Ethics and Health Care*, Philadelphia, Temple University Press, 1992, at pp.119–20

21. at p.120

22. Hammer, J. and Allen, P., 'Reproductive Engineering: The Final Solution?', in Birke, L. et al (eds), *Alice Through the Microscope*, London, Virago, 1980, 208, at p.222

23. Charlesworth, M., 'Human Genome Analysis and the Concept of Human Nature', in *Human Genetic Information: Science, Law and Ethics*, Ciba Foundation Symposium 149, Chichester, John Wiley & Sons, 1990, 180, at p.188

24. Corea, G., *The Mother Machine: Reproductive Technologies From Artificial Insemination to Artificial Wombs*, London, The Women's Press, 1988, at p.6

25. Corea, op.cit., at p.15

26. Rowland, op.cit., at p.6

27. Corea, op.cit., at p.169

28. Rowland, op.cit., at p.202

29. Foucault, M., *Madness and Civilisation: A History of Insanity in the Age of Reason*, London, Tavistock, 1967, at p.146

30. Schmidtke, J., 'Who Owns the Human Genome? Ethical and Legal Aspects', *J. Pharm. Pharmacol.* 44 (Suppl. 1), 205, at p.205

31. op.cit., at p.287

32. Corea, op.cit., at p.289

33. id.

34. Corea, op.cit., at p.4

35. Corea, op.cit., at p.3

36. op.cit., at p.129

37. Freely, M. and Pyper, C., *Pandora's Clock: Understanding Our Fertility*, London, Heinemann, 1993, at p.100

38. Corea, op.cit., at p.169
39. op.cit., at p.3
40. Human Fertilisation and Embryology Act 1990 s.13(5)
41. Human Reproductive Technology Bill s.23
42. Abortion Act 1967 (as amended)
43. Derived from *Roe* v. *Wade* 410 US 113 (1973). See for example, *Webster* v. *Reproductive Health Services* 492 US 490 (1989); *Planned Parenthood of Southeastern Pennsylvania* v. *Casey* 112 S Ct. 2791 (1992)
44. op.cit., at p.3
45. *R* v. *Ethical Committee of St. Mary's Hospital (Manchester)* ex parte *Harriott* [1988] 1 FLR 512
46. Swartz, M., 'Pregnant Woman vs Fetus: A Dilemma for Hospital Ethics Committees', 1 *Cambridge Quarterly of Healthcare Ethics* 51 (1992); Annas, G., 'Protecting the Liberty of Pregnant Patients', 316 *New England J. of Medicine* 1213 (1987); Purdy, L., 'Are Pregnant Women Fetal Containers?', Vol.4, No.4, Bioethics, 1990, 273. See also chapter 3, *infra*.
47. op.cit., at p.81
48. Sherwin, op.cit., at p.131
49. Hammer and Allen, loc.cit., at p.222
50. id.
51. op.cit., at p.6
52. c.f. Stanworth, M., 'Reproductive Technologies and the Deconstruction of Motherhood', in Stanworth, M. (ed) *Reproductive Technologies: Gender, Motherhood and Medicine*, Oxford, Polity Press, at p.17. 'The view of some feminists comes uncomfortably close to that espoused by some members of the medical professions. Infertile women are too easily 'blinded by science ...; they are manipulated into full and total support of any technique which will produce those desired children; the choices they make and even their motivations to choose are controlled by men; in this case it is the patriarchal and pronatal conditioning that makes infertile women (and by implication, all women) incapable of rationally grounded and authentic choice.'
53. Woollett, loc.cit., at p.171
54. See chapter 3, *infra*
55. For discussion of the use of this contraceptive product, see Vance, J.L., 'Womb for Rent: Norplant and the Undoing of Poor Women', 21(3)

Hastings Constitutional Law Quarterly 827 (1994); 'Long Acting Contraception: Moral Choices, Policy Dilemmas', *Hastings Center Report*, January-February 1995 (Special Supplement)

3 Women and Foetuses: Whose Rights?

An earlier version of this chapter was published as 'Moral Status (who or what counts?', in Bewley, S. and Ward, R.H. (eds), *Ethics in Obstetrics and Gynaecology, London*, RCOG Press, 1994. The material is reproduced by courtesy of the Royal College of Obstetricians and Gynaecologists.

1. Harrison, M.R., 'Unborn: Historical Perspective of the Foetus as a Patient', *The Pharos*, Winter 1982, 19, at pp.23–4
2. McCullogh, L.B. and Chervenak, F.A., *Ethics in Obstetrics and Gynaecology*, Oxford UP, 1994, at pp.100–1
3. Cm 9314/1984
4. para 11.9
5. Cm 762/1989
6. Mattingley, S.S., 'The Maternal-Fetal Dyad: Exploring the Two-Patient Model', Vol.22, No.1, *Hastings Center Report* (1992) 13, at p.14
7. Wells, C., 'Maternal Versus Foetal Rights', in Working Paper no.1, Feminist Legal Research Unit, University of Liverpool, 1992, 17, at pp.18–19
8. Johnsen, D., 'The Creation of Fetal Rights: Conflicts with Women's Constitutional Rights to Liberty, Privacy and Equal Protection', 95 *Yale Law Journal* (1986) 599, at p.599
9. *Hamilton* v. *Fife Health Board* [1993] 4 Med LR 201
10. Robertson, J. and Schulman, J., 'Pregnancy and Prenatal Harm to Offspring: The Case of Mothers with PKU', Vol.17, No.4, *Hastings Center Report*, 1987, 23, at p.32
11. op.cit., at p.102
12. *Hamilton*, supra cit.; *De Martell* v. *Merton and Sutton Health Authority* [1991] 2 Med LR 209; *B* v. *Islington Health Authority* [1991] 2 Med LR 133; *Montreal Tramways* v. *Leveille* [1933] 4 DLR 337; *Watt* v. *Rama* (unreported, Supreme Court of Victoria, Australia, 1972); *X and Y* v. *Pal and Others* [1992] 3 Med LR 195 (Court of Appeal, New South Wales)

13. Gregg, R., '"Choice" as a Double-Edged Sword: Information, Guilt and Mother-Blaming in a High-Tech Age', *Women and Health*, Vol. 20(3), 1993, 53, at p. 54

14, Gregg, loc.cit., at p. 55

15. McCullough and Chervenak, op.cit., at pp. 103–4

16. Ikenotos, L.C., 'Code of Perfect Pregnancy', *Ohio State Law Journal*, Vol. 33, 1992, 1205, at pp. 1293–4

17. Lew, J.B., 'Terminally Ill and Pregnant: State Denial of a Woman's Right to Refuse a Caesarian Section', *Buffalo Law Review*, Vol. 38, 1990, 619, at p. 642

18. Annas, G., 'Pregnant Women as Foetal Containers', Vol. 16, No. 6, *Hastings Center Report*, 1986, 13, at p. 14

19. c.f. *In re AC* 533 A.2d 611 (D.C.App. 1987); *Re AC* 573 A 2d 1235 (D.C. 1990) *Re S (Adult: Refusal of Medical Treatment)* [1992] 4 All ER 671. See also, *Jefferson v. Griffin Spaulding County Hospital Auth.* 247 Ga 274. For discussion of the issues raised by these kinds of decisions, see, e.g., Swartz, M., 'Pregnant Woman vs Foetus: A Dilemma for Hospital Ethics Committees', 1 *Cambridge Quarterly of Healthcare Ethics* 51 (1992); Johnsen, loc.cit.

20. op.cit., at pp. 103–4

21. Mattingley, loc.cit.

22. Beauchamp, T.L. and Childress, J.S., *Principles of Biomedical Ethics* (4th Ed.), Oxford UP, 1994

23. Annas, G., 'She's Going to Die: The Case of Angela C', Vol. 18, No. 1, *Hastings Center Report*, 1988, 23 at p. 24

24. loc.cit., at p. 621

25. loc.cit., at p. 56

26. Ruddick, W. and Wilcox, W., 'Operating on the Foetus', 12 *Hastings Center Report* 10 (1982), at p. 12

27. loc.cit., at p. 55

28. cf. *Re T (adult: refusal of medical treatment)* [1992] 4 All ER 649, where Lord Donaldson MR said at p. 653, the right exists 'notwithstanding that the reasons for making the choice are rational, irrational, unknown or even non-existent'; see also *Re C (adult: refusal of medical treatment)* [1994] 1 All ER 819 where the court endorsed the right of a man suffering from paranoid schizophrenia to refuse life-saving treatment.

29. Purdy, L., 'Are Pregnant Women Foetal Containers?', Vol. 4, No. 4,

Bioethics, 1990, 273, at p.273

30. Annas, G., 'Protecting the Liberty of Pregnant Patients', 316 *New England J. of Medicine*, 1213 (1987), at p.1213
31. see note 19, supra
32. loc.cit., at p.622
33. id.
34. Annas, loc.cit. (1988), at p.25
35. loc.cit., at p.627
36. *Re S*, supra cit.
37. *Re C* and *Re W*, reported in *The Times* and the *Guardian* 16 September 1996
38. *Re AC* 573 A 2d 1235 (D.C.1990) at p.1248
39. id.
40. Draper, H., 'Women, Forced Caesarians and Antenatal Responsibilities', *Working Paper No.1*, Feminist Legal Research Unit, University of Liverpool, 1992, at p.12
41. Review of the Guidance on the Research Use of Foetuses and Foetal Material, Cm 762/1989
42. loc.cit., at p.1266
43. Bayer, R., 'Women, Work and Reproductive Hazards', 12 *Hastings Center Report*, 14 (1982)
44. loc.cit., at p.1241
45. at p.1286
46. Ikenotos, loc.cit., at p.1244
47. loc.cit., at p.1259
48. Cook, R.J. and Plata, M.I., 'Women's reproductive rights', *International Journal of Gynecology and Obstetrics* 44 (1994) 215, at p.218
49. loc.cit., at p.613

4 A Woman's Right to Choose?: Law, Medicine and Abortion

1. Dworkin, R., *Life's Dominion: An Argument about Abortion and Euthanasia*, London, HarperCollins, 1993, at p.4
2. Luker, K., *Abortion and the Politics of Motherhood*, University of California Press, 1984, at p.12
3. For further discussion, see McLean, S.A.M., and Britton, A., *The*

Case for Physician Assisted Suicide, London, Pandora Press, 1997

4. op.cit., at p.93
5. Luker, op.cit., at p.93
6. Mohr, J., *Abortion in America*, OUP, 1979
7. at p.162
8. McLaren, A., *Birth Control in Nineteenth-Century England*, London, Croom Helm, 1978, at p.240
9. Petersen, K., *Abortion Regimes*, Aldershot, Dartmouth, 1993, at p.49
10. Jackson, S., et al (eds), *Women's Studies: A Reader*, Hemel Hempstead, Harvester Wheatsheaf, 1993, at p.365
11. op.cit., at p.66
12. *R* v. *Bourne* [1939] 1 KB 687
13. Rowbotham, S., *Hidden From History*, Pluto Press, 1973
14. at p.155
15. Luker, op.cit., at p.109
16. op.cit., at p.101
17. Wikler, N.J., 'Society's Response to the New Reproductive Technologies: The Feminist Perspectives', *Southern California Law Review*, Vol.59:1043 (1986), at p.1049
18. op.cit., at p.57
19. op.cit., at p.364
20. *Roe* v. *Wade* 410 US 113 (1973)
21. at p.164
22. c.f. *Thornburgh* v. *American College of Obstetricians and Gynecologists* 476 US 747 (1986); *Webster* v. *Reproductive Health Services* 492 US 490 (1989); *Ohio* v. *Akron Center for Reproductive Health* 497 US 502 (1990); *Planned Parenthood of Southeastern Pennsylvania* v. *Casey* 112 S Ct. 2791 (1992)
23. Quoted in Ginsburg, R.B., '*Roe* v. *Wade*', *North Carolina Law Review*, Vol. 63, 1985, 375, at p.381
24. loc. cit., at p.382
25. at p.375
26. at p.383
27. at p.385
28. loc.cit., at p.171
29. For further discussion, see chapter 8, infra
30. op.cit., at p.185

31. at p.245

32. Rothman, B.K., 'The products of conception: The social context of reproductive choices', *Journal of Medical Ethics*, 1985, 11, 188, at p.189

33. Human Fertilisation and Embryology Act 1990 amending the Abortion Act 1967. The relevant section is s.1(1)(d) if '... there is a substantial risk that if the child were born it would suffer from such physical or mental abnormalities as to be seriously disabled.'

34. Furedi, A., *The Progress Guide to Preimplantation Diagnosis*, Progress Educational Trust Publication, at p.3

35. id.

36. Hubbard, R. and Wald, E., *Exploding the Gene Myth*, Boston, Beacon Press, 1993, at p.30

37. op.cit., at p.28

38. op.cit.

39. Dworkin, op.cit., particularly at p.57, where he says: 'It is true that many women's attitudes toward abortion are affected by a contradictory sense of both identification with and oppression by their pregnancies, and that the sexual, economic, and social subordination of women contributes to that undermining sense of oppression. In a better society, which supported child rearing as enthusiastically as it discourages abortion, the status of a foetus probably would change, because women's sense of pregnancy and motherhood as creative would be more genuine and less compromised, and the inherent value of their own lives less threatened.'

5 Controlling Fertility: The Case of Mentally Disabled People

1. Lee, R. and Morgan, D., 'A Lesser Sacrifice? Sterilisation and Mentally Handicapped Women', in Lee, R. and Morgan, D. (eds), *Birthrights: Law and Ethics at the Beginning of Life*, London, Routledge, 1990, at p.132

2. Shaw, J., 'Sterilisation of Mentally Handicapped People: Judges Rule OK?', 53 *Modern Law Review*, 91, 1990, at pp.102–3

3. *Sterilisation*, Law Reform Commission of Canada, Working Paper 24 (1979), at p.50

4. *Re Eve* 31 DLR (4th) 1, 1987

5. at p.31
6. Universal Declaration of Human Rights 1948, Article 16 says 'Men and women of full age ... have the right to marry and found a family.'
7. European Convention on Human Rights 1950 (entered into force 3 September 1953) Article 12 says 'Men and women of marriageable age have the right to marry and to found a family, according to the national laws governing the exercise of this right.'
8. Per La Forest, J., in *Re Eve*, supra cit., at p.34
9. *Re Eve*, at p.29
10. *Lawrence, Petitioner* 32 BMLR 87 (1996)
11. Re D (a minor) [1976] 1 All ER 326
12. supra cit.
13. at p.332
14. at pp.334–5
15. at p.9
16. at p.32
17. Shaw, loc.cit., at p.91
18. For further discussion, see McLean, S.A.M., 'The Right to Reproduce', in Campbell, et al. (eds), *Human Rights: From Rhetoric to Reality*, Oxford, Basil Blackwell, 1986
19. 274 US 200 (1927)
20. at p.207
21. 316 US 535 (1942)
22. at p.541
23. Norrie, K. McK., *Family Planning Practice and the Law*, Aldershot, Dartmouth, 1991, at p.109
24. Dickens, B., 'Retardation and Sterilisation' 5, *Int. J. Law Psy* 295 (1983), at p.316
25. [1989] 2 All ER 545
26. loc.cit., p.98
27. *Re Eve*, supra cit., at p.31
28. (1981) 85 NJ 235
29. loc.cit.
30. id.
31. per La Forest, J., in *Re Eve*, supra cit., at p.27
32. Mason, J.K., *Medico-Legal Aspects of Reproduction and Parenthood*, Aldershot, Dartmouth, 1990

33. (1980) 73 Wn 2d 228

34. supra cit.

35. *Re Guardianship of Tully* (1978) 146 Cal.Rptr. 266 (C.A.)

36. at p.270

37. (1981) 307 N.W. 2d 881 (Wis. S.C.)

38. at p.895

39. Norrie, op.cit., at p.120

40. supra cit.

41. (1985) 19 DLR (4th) 255

42. per Anderson, J.A., at p.275

43. *Re Eve*, supra cit., at p.34

44. *F* v. *Berkshire Health Authority*, supra cit., at p.551

45. Ogbourne, D. and Ward, R., 'The Mentally Incompetent and the Courts', *Anglo-American Law Review*, 18, 230 (1989), at p.235

46. *Re B (A Minor)(Wardship: Sterilisation)* [1987] 2 All ER 206 (HL)

47. at p.1217

48. [1987] 2 All ER 206

49. At pp.210–11

50. at p.219

51. derived from the case of *Bolam* v. *Friern Hospital Management Committee* [1957] 2 All ER 118

52. loc.cit., at p.236

53. Brazier, M., 'Sterilisation: Down the Slippery Slope?', *Professional Negligence*, March 1990, 25, at p.27

54. *Re M (A Minor)(Wardship: Sterilisation)* [1988] 2 FLR 997

55. *Re P (A Minor)(Wardship: Sterilisation)* [1989] 1 FLR 182

56. loc.cit., at p.26

57. loc.cit., at p.27

58. supra cit., at p.91

59. Freeman, M.D.A., 'For Her Own Good', *The Law Society's Gazette*, Wednesday 1 April 1987, 949

60. at p.949

61. Gillon, R., 'On Sterilising Severely Mentally Handicapped People', *Journal of Medical Ethics*, 1987, 13

62. Brazier, loc.cit., at p.26

6 The Infant with Disability: To Treat or Not to Treat?

1. Smith, S.R., 'Disabled Newborns and the Federal Child Abuse Amendments: Tenuous Protection', *The Hastings Law Journal*, Vol. 37, May 1986, 765, at pp.767–8

2. Wells, C., 'Whose Baby Is It?', *J. Law and Society*, Vol. 15, No.4, 1988, 323, at p.325

3. Shapiro, R., 'Medical Treatment of Defective Newborns: An Answer to the "Baby Doe" Dilemma', *Harvard Journal on Legislation*, Vol. 20:137 (1983), at p.147

4. Whitelaw, A., 'Death as an Option in Neonatal Intensive Care', *The Lancet*, August 9, 1986, 328, at p.328

5. Campbell, A.G.M. and Duff, R.S., 'Deciding the Care of Severely Malformed or Dying Infants', *Journal of Medical Ethics*, 1979, 5, 65, at p.65

6. Robertson, J.A., 'Involuntary Euthanasia of Defective Newborns: A Legal Analysis', *Stanford Law Review*, Vol. 27:213 (1975), at p.268

7. Mason, J.K., *Medico-Legal Aspects of Reproduction and Parenthood*, Aldershot, Dartmouth, 1990, at p.251

8. Post, S.G., 'History, Infanticide and Imperiled Newborns', *Hastings Center Report*, Vol. 18 no.4, 1988, 14, at p.17

9. Smith, loc.cit., at p.785

10. McLean, S.A.M. and Maher, G., *Medicine, Morals and the Law*, Aldershot, Gower, 1983 (reprinted 1985), at p.62

11. at pp.62–3

12. Mason, op.cit., at p.263

13. Smith, loc.cit., at pp.768–9

14. Rhoden, N., 'Treatment Dilemmas for Imperiled Newborns: Why Quality of Life Counts', *Southern California Law Review*, Vol. 58, 1985, 1283, at p.1331

15. Williams, G., 'Down's Syndrome and the Duty to Preserve Life', *New Law Journal*, October 1, 1981, 1020

16. at p.1021

17. loc.cit., at p.770

18. Simply put, the doctrine countenances a bad side-effect coming from an otherwise good act as being morally acceptable so long as it was not intended. This was accepted into English law by the case of *R* v.

Adams [1957] Crim. L.R. 365

19. Rhoden, loc.cit., at p.1347

20. id.

21. cf. Glover, J., *Causing Death and Saving Lives*, Harmondsworth, Penguin, 1977 (reprinted 1984)

22. Kuhse, H. and Singer, P., 'For Sometimes Letting- and Helping-Die', Vol 14, No. 3–4, *Law, Medicine and Health Care*, 149, at p.151

23. id.

24. op.cit.

25. loc.cit., at p.15

26. id.

27. Templeman, L. J., in *Re B (A Minor)(Wardship: Medical Treatment)* (1981) [1990] 3 All ER 927, at p.929

28. Wells, loc.cit., at p.323

29. Smith, loc.cit., at pp.768–9

30. loc.cit., at pp.214–15

31. McLean and Maher, op.cit., at p.70

32. Blank, R.H., 'Treatment of Critically Ill Newborns in Australasia', *The Journal of Legal Medicine*, 16:211 (1995) at p.221

33. *Re F; F v. Supreme Court of Victoria*, 2 July 1986 (unreported)

34. id.

35. *R v. Arthur* (1981) 12 BMLR 1

36. at p.22

37. Ellis, T.S., 'Letting Defective Babies Die: Who Decides?' *American Journal of Law and Medicine*, Vol.7 No. 4, 393, at p.415

38. loc.cit., at p.153

39. Phillips, P.M., 'Treatment Decisions for Seriously Ill Newborns: Who Should Decide?', *Capital University Law Review*, 21, 919 (1992), at p.921

40. 321 US 158 (1944)

41. at p.170

42. 406 US 205 (1972)

43. at pp.233–4

44. loc.cit., at p.777

45. *Re B*, supra cit., at p.1422

46. Record of Investigation of Death, Case No. 3149/89, 29 October 1991, at p.30, quoted in Blank, loc.cit.

47. loc.cit., at p.214

48. at p.216

49. Raphael, D.D., 'Handicapped Infants: Medical Ethics and the Law', *Journal of Medical Ethics*, 1988, 14, 5, at p.6

50. Smith, loc.cit., at p.783

51. loc.cit., at p.953

52. loc.cit., at p.1343

53. id.

54. loc.cit., at p.245

55. loc.cit., at p.960

56. loc.cit., at p.66

57. id.

58. loc.cit., at p.331

59. 379 So. 2d 359 (Fla. 1980) where it was said at p.360 that because the decision about withholding/withdrawing treatment (in this case not from a baby) was complex 'and encompasses the interests of the law, both civil and criminal, medical ethics and social morality, it is not one which is well-suited for resolution in any adversary judicial proceeding.'

60. loc.cit., at p.216

61. loc.cit., at p.7

62. Rhoden, loc.cit., at p.1322

63. Wells, loc.cit., at p.336

64. id.

65. *In the Matter of Baby "K"* 16 F. 3d 590 (1994)

66. Phillips, loc.cit., at p.956

67. Smith, loc.cit., at p.778

68. Robertson, loc.cit., at p.266

69. Phillips, loc.cit., at p.962

7 Choosing Life or Death

1. Capron, A., 'Legal and Ethical Problems in Decisions for Death', *Law, Medicine and Health Care*, Vol.14, No. 3–4, 1986, 141, at p.141

2. Illich, I., *Limits to Medicine. Medical Nemesis:The Expropriation of Health*, Harmondsworth, Penguin, 1977, at p.179

3. Kass, L.R., *Toward a More Natural Science: Biology and Human Affairs*, New York, The Free Press, 1985, at p.20

4. For discussion, see McLean S.A.M. and Britton, A., *The Case for Physician Assisted Suicide*, London, Pandora, 1997

5. op.cit., at p.158

6. Illich, op.cit., at p.244

7. *Guidelines on the Termination of Life-Sustaining Treatment and the Care of the Dying*, Report by the Hastings Center, 1987, p.viii

8. Kass, op.cit., at p.32

9. loc.cit., at p.143

10. *Re T* (adult: refusal of medical treatment) [1992] 3 Med LR 306, at p.314

11. Angell, M., 'Prisoners of Technology: The Case of Nancy Cruzan', 322 *New England J. of Medicine*, 1226 (1990), at p.1228

12. For further discussion, see McLean and Britton, op.cit.

13. Annas, G.J., 'Nancy Cruzan in China' 20 *Hastings Center Report*, Sept/Oct 1990, 39, at p.39

14. Shepard, R.T., 'Family Decisionmaking and Foregoing Treatment: A Judicial Perspective', *Issues in Law & Medicine*, Vol.10 No 3, 1994, 251, at p.251

15. Weir, R.S., 'The Morality of Physician-Assisted Suicide', *Law Medicine & Health Care*, Vol.20, 1–2, Spring-Summer, 1992, 116, at p.116

16. loc.cit., at p.144

17. Capron, loc.cit., at p.141

18. Kuhse, H., 'The Case for Active Voluntary Euthanasia', *Law, Medicine & Health Care*, Vol.14, No. 3–4, 1986, at p. 145

19. *Airedale NHS Trust* v. *Bland* [1993] 2 W.L.R. 359, per Lord Browne-Wilkinson at p.382

20. At p.387

21. Capron, loc.cit., at p.142

22. For discussion, see Beauchamp, T.L. and Childress, J.S., *Principles of Biomedical Ethics*, (4th edn) Oxford UP, 1994.

23. [1993] 4 Med LR 239

24. at p. 247

25. McLean, S.A.M., 'Law at the End of Life: What Next?', in McLean, S.A.M.(ed.), *Death, Dying and the Law*, Aldershot, Dartmouth, 1996, at p.63

26. at p.243
27. cf. *Re Quinlan* 355 A 2d 664 (N.J., 1976); *Cruzan* v. *Missouri Department of Health* 110 S Ct 2841 (1990)
28. Capron, loc.cit., at p.143
29. *Airedale NHS Trust* v. *Bland*, supra cit., per Lord Goff, at p.367
30. per Lord Keith, at p.363
31. Lord Mustill, at p.398, 'The distressing truth which must not be shirked is that the proposed conduct is not in the best interests of Anthony Bland, for he has no best interests of any kind.'
32. c.f. McLean, S.A.M., *A Patient's Right to Know: Information Disclosure, the Doctor and The Law*, Aldershot, Dartmouth, 1989
33. per Lord Goff, at p.372
34. American Medical Association Council on Ethical and Judicial Affairs, *Withholding or Withdrawing Life-prolonging Medical Treatment*, JAMA 1986;236:471; American Medical Association Council on Scientific Affairs, *Persistent Vegetative State and the Decision to Withdraw or Withhold Life Support*, JAMA 1990; 263: 426
35. *Auckland Health Board* v. *Attorney General*, supra cit., at p.249
36. at p.369
37. id.
38. op.cit., at p.225
39. Rachels, J., *At the End of Life: Euthanasia and Morality*, Oxford UP, 1986, at p.148
40. at p.388
41. id.
42. pp.388–9
43. At p.387
44. id.
45. McLean, loc.cit., at p.61
46. McLean, loc.cit., at p.58
47. 385 SE 2d 651 (Ga., 1989)
48. Fletcher, J., *Morals and Medicine*, Princeton University Press, 1954, at p.227
49. id.
50. Fletcher, J., 'The Courts and Euthanasia', *Law, Medicine & Health Care*, Volume 15:4, Winter 1987/88, 223, at p.226
51. *Rodriguez* v. *British Columbia* [1993] S.C.J. No 94 (September 30,

1993)

52. Death With Dignity Act 1994 (now referred to as Oregon Measure 16 of 1994)

53. *Lee* v. *State of Oregon* (1995) Civil No. 94–6467–Ho.D. Ore. August 3

54. *Quill* v. *Vacco* F. 3d (2nd Cir. 1996) No. 95-7028

55. *Quill* v. *Vacco: Compassion in Dying (Glucksberg)* v. *Washington* 117 S.Ct 2293 (1997)

56. Lord Mustill, in *Airedale NHS Trust* v. *Bland*, supra cit.at p.391

57. Fletcher, loc.cit. (1987/88), at p.225

58. Harris Poll No.9, 1995, released 30 January 1995

59. For discussion, see McLean, S.A.M. and Britton, A., *Sometimes a Small Victory*, published by the Institute of Law and Ethics in Medicine, Glasgow University, 1996 (printed by Scottish Country Press), Appendix 3

60. Kirby, M., 'Bioethics '89: Can Democracy Cope?', 18, 1–2 Spring/Summer 1990, *Law, Medicine & Health Care*, 5, at p.6

8 Controlling or Conceding the Future?

1. Have, H., 'Physicians' Priorities – Patients' Expectations', in Szawarski, Z. and Evans, D. (eds), *Solidarity, Justice and Health Care Priorities, Linkoping*, LCC, Linkoping University, 1993, 42, at p.43

2. Callahan, D., *What Kind of Life:The Limits of Medical Progress*, New York, Simon and Schuster, 1990, at p.25.

3. For further discussion, see McLean, S.A.M. and Britton, A., *The Case for Physician Assisted Suicide*, London, Pandora Press, 1997

4. c.f. Wilkie, T., *Perilous Knowledge: The Human Genome Project and its Implications*, London, Faber and Faber, 1993; McLean, S.A.M., 'Mapping the Human Genome — Friend or Foe?', *Soc.Sci.Med.* Vol.39, No.9, 1221; McLean, S.A.M., 'The New Genetics: A Challenge to Clinical Values?', *Proc. R. Coll. Physicians*, Edinburgh 1996; 26: 41; McLean, S.A.M., 'Science's "Holy Grail" — Some Legal and Ethical Implications of the Human Genome Project', in Freeman, M.D.A. (ed.) *Current Legal Problems* (1995) Vol.48 Part II, Oxford UP, 233

5. United States Department of Energy, Office of Energy Research Office of Environmental Research, Human Genome 1991–92 Program

Report (Washington, DC 1992), iii

6. Robinson, A., 'The Ethics of Gene Research', *Can. Med. Assoc. J.*, 1994: 150(5) 721, at p.721

7. *Our Genetic Future: The Science and Ethics of Genetic Technology*, OUP, 1992, at p.1

8. Maddox, J., 'The Case for the Human Genome', *Nature*, Vol.352, 4 July 1991, 11, at p.12

9. Galloway, J., 'Britain and the Human Genome', *New Scientist*, 26 July 1990, 25, at p.25

10. Murray, T.H., 'Ethical Issues in Human Genome Research', *The FASEB Journal*, Vol.5, January 1991, at p.55

11. BMA, op.cit., at p.4

12. *Ethical Issues in Clinical Genetics,* Royal College of Physicians of London, 1991, p.4, para 3.1

13. BMA, op.cit., at p.172

14. Schmidtke, J., 'Who Owns the Human Genome?' *Ethical and Legal Aspects, J. Pharm. Pharmacol.*, 44 (Suppl. 1) 205, at pp.205–6.

15. Engelhardt, H.T., *The Foundation of Bioethics*, New York, OUP, 1986, at p.181

16. Maddox, J., 'New Genetics Means No New Ethics', *Nature*, Vol.364, 8 July 1993, at p.97

17. Fletcher, J.C. and Wertz, D.C., 'An International Code of Ethics in Medical Genetics Before the Human Genome is Mapped', in Bankowski, Z. and Capron, A. (eds), *Genetics, Ethics and Human Values: Human Genome Mapping, Genetic Screening and Therapy*, xxiv CIOMS Round Table Conference, at p.97

18. op.cit., at p.182

19. Davis, J., 'Ethical Issues', in Ryan, M.P., et al, 'Genetic Testing for Familial Hypertrophic Cardiomyopathy in Newborn Infants', *BMJ* 1992, 310, at p.858

20. Hubbard, R. and Wald, E., *Exploding the Gene Myth*, Boston, Beacon Press, 1993, at p.30

21. Furedi, A., *The Progress Guide to Preimplantation Diagnosis, A Progress Educational Trust Publication*, at p.3

22. op.cit., at p.30

23. id.

24. Skene, L., 'Mapping the Human Genome: Some Thoughts for those

Who Say "There Should be a Law on It"', *Bioethics*, Vol. 5, No. 3, 1991, 233, at p. 238

25. Charlesworth, M., 'Human Genome Analysis and the Concept of Human Nature', in *Ciba Foundation Symposium*, no. 149, Chichester, John Wiley & Sons, 1990, at p. 188

26. Davis, B.D., 'Limits to Genetic Intervention in Humans: Somatic and Germline', in *Ciba Foundation Symposium*, supra cit., 81, at pp. 83–4

27. This has since been extended

28. *Human Genome News*, 'Insurance Task Force Makes Recommendations', Vol. 5, No. 2, July 1993, at p. 1

29. House of Commons Science and Technology Committee, *Third Report, Human Genetics: The Science and its Consequences*, London, HMSO, Paper 41–1

30. Nuffield Council on Bioethics, *Genetic Screening: Ethical Issues*, London, 1993, p. 61, para 6.20

31. Murray, loc. cit., at p. 56

32. op. cit., at p. 214

33. Charlesworth, loc. cit., at p. 180

34. Rose, S., Kamin, L., Lewontin, R., *Not in our Genes: Biology, Ideology and Human Nature*, Harmondsworth, Penguin, 1984, at p. 10

35. Hubbard and Wald, op. cit., at p. 36

36. op. cit., at p. 137

37. Davis, Ciba Foundation, supra cit., at p. 86

38. Brahams, D., 'Human Genetic Information: The Legal Implications', in *Ciba Foundation Symposium*, 11, at p. 117

39. loc. cit., at p. 205

40. Koehn, D., *The Ground of Professional Ethics*, London, Routledge, 1994, 180

41. Miller, J., *The Body in Question*, Bookclub Associates by arrangement with Jonathan Cape Ltd., London, 1980, at p. 52

Index